THE FAR-REACHING BENEF

Infant massage, as it is shared in this *that connects you deeply with the person who is your baby, and it helps you to understand your baby's particular nonverbal language and respond with love and respectful listening. It empowers you as a parent, for it gives you the means by which you become an expert on your own child and therefore can respond according to your baby's unique needs. Rather than growing up selfish and demanding (though all kids go through such stages), a child whose voice is heard, whose heart is full, and who is enveloped in love overflows with that love and naturally, unselfconsciously gives of himself to others. He learns what healthy, respectful touch is by being touched that way. He learns self-discipline by watching his parents and imitating them. The deep emotional bonds formed in infancy lay a foundation for a lifetime of trust, courage, dependability, faith, and love.*

"Vimala McClure is a visionary who has helped innumerable people become far better parents. She has become my own personal Dr. Spock: the main source I turn to for loving and competent guidance and inspiration in raising my children."

—Marc Allen, author of *Visionary Business* and *A Visionary Life*

"What a brilliant way to love and nurture a child! The first connection between parent and child is physical, through the body; by using the techniques that Vimala has developed, your parental relationship will be off to a magnificent start."

—Judy Ford, author of *Wonderful Ways to Love a Child* and *Wonderful Ways to Be a Family*

"Embodying spirit is the work of our times...and the beautiful, empowering words of Vimala McClure bring to our everyday life a deep and abiding experience of the timeliness of the body, soul, and spirit. We are changed."

—Carolyn Craft, director of WISDOM Radio

Other books by Vimala McClure

A Woman's Guide to Tantra Yoga

The Tao of Motherhood

Bangladesh: Rivers in a Crowded Land

The Path of Parenting: Twelve Principles to Guide Your Journey

Teaching Infant Massage: A Handbook for Instructors

Infant Massage

A Handbook for Loving Parents

VIMALA MCCLURE

THIRD REVISED EDITION

BANTAM BOOKS

New York Toronto London Sydney Auckland

INFANT MASSAGE: A HANDBOOK FOR LOVING PARENTS

PUBLISHING HISTORY
Originally published by Monterey Laboratories, Inc.
Portions of chapters ten and twelve previously appeared in
Mothering Magazine (Summer '86 and Spring '87)
Bantam Books trade paperback published September 1982
Revised Bantam edition published September 1989
Third revised Bantam edition/November 2000
Photograph on page 190 appeared in original 1982 edition.

Book design by Virginia Norey.

Library of Congress Cataloging-in-Publication Data
McClure, Vimala Schneider, 1952–
    Infant massage : a handbook for loving parents / by Vimala
McClure.—3rd rev. ed.
        p. cm.
    Includes bibliographical references and index.
    ISBN 0-553-38056-7
    1. Massage for infants—Handbooks, manuals, etc.   I. Title.

RJ61 .M48 2000
649'.4—dc21   00-039754

Published simultaneously in the United States and Canada

Bantam Books are published by Bantam Books, a division of Random
House, Inc. Its trademark, consisting of the words "Bantam Books" and the
portrayal of a rooster, is Registered in U.S. Patent and Trademark Office
and in other countries. Marca Registrada. Bantam Books, 1540 Broadway,
New York, New York 10036.

PRINTED IN THE UNITED STATES OF AMERICA

12 14 16 18 20 19 17 15 13

Dedicated to
P. R. Sarkar
and to my beloved children

Frail newborn wings,
Small voice that sings,
New little beating heart,
Dread not thy birth,
Nor fear the earth—
The Infinite thou art.
The sun doth shine
The earth doth spin,
For welcome—enter in
This green and daisied sphere.
Rejoice—and have no fear.

—Richard LeGallienne

CONTENTS

ACKNOWLEDGMENTS

HEARTFELT THANKS TO all those who have helped and supported my work over the years. Special thanks to the following people for helping bring this new edition to birth: to Toni Burbank and Robin Michaelson for making it happen; to all the trainers in the International Association of Infant Massage (IAIM) for their input, experience, and support; to Peggy O'Mara, founder and publisher of *Mothering Magazine*, who started her work just about the time I did and has been a great inspiration to me all these years.

I thank my friends and colleagues in the International Association of Infant Massage for their hard work, dedication, and service to humanity through this work. It is their realization of its long-range potential that has brought its benefits to so many parents worldwide and, I believe, contributed to a significant change in our infant parenting practices and the way we respond to infants' needs.

A huge thank you to trainer Clara Ute Zacher Laves and her husband Markus Zacher, and also to infant massage instructor Joni Rubenstein and her teen parents for helping get the new photographs done and being so conscientious in doing so.

I also want to acknowledge my sister Madhi Shirman, whose encouragement supported me to begin teaching infant massage in the first place, and whose unwavering support of my work has meant the world to me.

The photographer who took the beautiful photos in Chapter 8 as well as some others is Günter Kiepke. Thank you, Günter; you did the most wonderful job and far exceeded my expectations!

In the process of putting this book together, I used many, many photos and was unable to use three times the final choices. I want to thank all the parents and babies who allowed me to photograph them or have other photographers do it for me. I may accidentally leave out a name in the following list, if the photos were taken elsewhere and I can't find the name, or so long ago I can't remember which release goes with which name. But please know I am very grateful to everyone who contributed in any way; by doing so, you have contributed to the well-being of future generations.

The people who graciously allowed me to use their photographs (which may or may not appear in this book):

—Maraliz Bracamonte, Naidelyn Alvarez
—Andrea Bassett, Deondre Beckwith
—Bridgett Washington, Allezae Brown
—Gabriel De La Luz, Christina Hogbin, Gabriel De La Luz Jr.
—Shenika Evans, Shavel Evans
—Yvette Hernandez, Julette Contreras
—Alexandria Boney
—Anke D. Bahr, Lenja Kim
—Oliver Fuchs
—Corinna Reissner, Anna Catharina
—Susan Whittlesey, Anne Young
—Nancy Duffy, Nicole Green
—Susan Pressel, Justin Pressel
—Marlene Stieha, Analeesa Stieha
—Gina Kincaid, Elaina Marie Santa Cruz
—Yvonne Ruiz, Ashley Rodriguez
—Cindy Shelton, Christina Shelton
—Jan Lapetino and baby
—Heidi Dorsey, Tia Dorsey, Carlos Dorsey
—Mary Foster, Lance Foster, Michael Foster
—Clara Ute Zacher Laves
—Gabriela Silva, Jasline Ariana Garcia

FOREWORD

A GIFT OF TOUCH

IN THE SUMMER OF 1974, when my first child was born, I didn't
know anything about infant massage, but I knew that I wanted to
touch my baby. It was a hot summer, and it felt good to carry my
daughter around skin to skin. I would take her outside and lay her
on a blanket in the fresh air under the eaves of our house. There I
would rub her with sweet almond oil and massage her soft skin.

At about this same time, a few hundred miles away, Vimala was
massaging her babies. Vimala is the premier proponent of infant
massage in the world and was among the first to write about massage in general and infant massage in particular. In fact, Vimala's
work in infant massage has been instrumental in the birth of touch
therapy and bodywork in the United States and has helped to pop-
ularize and legitimize massage throughout the world. Her early
work on infant massage and premature babies was years ahead of its
time and continues to influence the humane care of newborns
through touch.

For many of us, infant massage has been a way to learn to touch
our babies and to become comfortable with touch in general. Those
of us who became parents in the 1960s and 1970s grew up in much
less intimate and "touchy-feely" times than today. Seeing people
hugging affectionately in public as we do today was almost unheard
of twenty years ago, when Vimala's innocent book sparked a revolution in touch in the United States.

As revolutionary as it is, infant massage is really an old-fashioned idea, and its beauty lies in the fact that anyone can do it. It's simple and it's good for you. It can't hurt you or your baby and it costs nothing. Don't think that you need special skills or talents to massage your baby. It comes naturally and is a way for our babies to teach us about themselves and for us to learn how to touch.

Touch is as necessary to the human baby as is food. Anthropologist Margaret Mead studied tribal societies all over the world and found that the most violent tribes were those that withheld touch in infancy. Neurologist Richard Restak says that physically holding and carrying an infant turn out to be the most important factors responsible for the infant's normal mental and social development. The effects of this normal development do not just influence infancy but impact the neural and neuroendocrine functions underlying emotional behavior in enduring ways. In other words, the more we experience authentic intimacy as infants, the more we are capable of intimacy as adults. And what can be more intimate than gentle touch?

Research at the University of Miami School of Medicine suggests that massage can stimulate nerves in the brain that facilitate food absorption, resulting in faster weight gain. Massage can lower stress hormones, resulting in improved immune function. Touch therapy can also help premature infants gain weight faster, asthmatic children improve breathing function, diabetic children comply with treatment, and sleepless babies fall asleep more easily. Other research indicates that touch therapy can benefit infants and children with eczema and can improve parent-baby interactions.

What better way to improve parent-baby interactions, what better way to ensure your baby is getting enough skin-to-skin contact, than with infant massage? The soothing oil and the soft easy touch of your hands are sensory delights that you can share with your baby as you introduce him to the world. Massage is such a nice way to get to know your baby and to spend time together in the early weeks and months. Soon enough she will be up and around, and these touch times of the early months will be sweet memories.

It was eight years between those first "massages" I gave my

daughter and the first real massage I had myself. It was not until the 1980s that massage therapists were easily available, and it took me many years to become comfortable with the idea of "indulging" in massage. Something that at first seemed frivolous to me has now become a cornerstone of my health care. Vimala has taught us that touch is not a self-indulgence but is actually a basic human need. How unfortunate that we would consider fulfilling such a basic need to be self-indulgent.

I would recommend that you spoil your children with the indulgence of your touch. Perhaps there is nothing quite so personal and intimate as the gift of infant massage. Like parenthood in general, infant massage enriches the parent as well as the baby. It establishes a tradition of touch that will enhance your relationship with your child for years to come.

Peggy O'Mara
Editor and Publisher
Mothering Magazine

PREFACE

❦

D URING THE PAST THREE DECADES, physicians have reassessed the importance of maternal-infant bonding in relation to development. Studies conducted at the University of Colorado and elsewhere have demonstrated that infants whose mothers have difficulty in touching, cuddling, or talking to them during the first few months of life are more likely to suffer from developmental growth or delay. Scientific advances in the understanding of the newborn and infant sensory, motor, and cognitive processes have resulted in new appreciation for many of the cultural parenting practices of the nonindustrialized world. For example, infant carrier packs such as the Snugli are modeled after practices observed in many parts of Africa and Latin America. These infant carriers promote mutual feelings of comfort and security associated with close body contact and still provide the parent freedom of movement.

In *Infant Massage: A Handbook for Loving Parents*, Vimala McClure introduces us to a form of parenting that has been practiced for centuries in India. The value of infant massage as a parenting technique can be appreciated best by recognizing the maternal-infant interaction as displayed in the faces of parents and babies shown in the pictures in this book. Hopefully, parents will accept infant massage into the American way of life in the same way that Lamaze childbirth classes and infant carriers have been accepted. An added plus to infant massage is the opportunity it provides for the father, especially of a breastfed baby, to have positive interaction with his child.

As a pediatrician, the best advice I can give you is to try the techniques described in this book. If the interaction between you and your child is enjoyable and the massage is fun, you will be providing your infant with a pleasurable form of stimulation that may build a strong foundation for your child's development.

Stephen Berman, M.D., F.A.A.P.
President, American Academy of Pediatrics
Chief of General Pediatrics
University of Colorado School of Medicine
and the Children's Hospital

INTRODUCTION

W HILE STUDYING AND WORKING in a small orphanage in India in 1973, I made a discovery that was to substantially redirect my life.

I became aware of the importance of traditional Indian baby massage, both for its soothing effects and for its role in affectionate nonverbal communication. An Indian mother regularly massages everyone in her family and passes these techniques on to her daughters. At the orphanage, the eldest massaged the little ones nearly every day. It was a type of nurturing I hadn't seen in the United States. I received its benefits when, during my last week in India, I succumbed to malaria. When I was delirious with fever, all the women in the neighborhood came to look after me. They massaged my body with practiced hands, as if I were a baby, and they sang to me, taking turns until my fever broke. I will never forget the feeling of their hands and hearts touching me.

On my way to the train station after a tearful good-bye at the orphanage, my rickshaw stopped to let a buffalo cart go by. To my right was a shanty—just a few boards and some canvas—where a family lived by the road. A young mother sat in the dirt with her baby across her knees, lovingly massaging him and singing. As I watched her, I thought, *There is so much more to life than material wealth.* She had so little, yet she could offer her baby this beautiful gift of love and security, a gift that would help to make him a compassionate human being.

I thought about all the children I had known in India, and how loving, warm, and playful they were in spite of their so-called disadvantages. They took care of one another, and they accepted responsibility without reservation. Perhaps, I thought, they are able to be so loving, so relaxed and natural because they have been loved like this as infants, and infants have been loved this way in India for thousands of years. Massage, perhaps, makes them at home in their world, not enemies or conquerors of it. It welcomes them to the warmth and love that is here for them, allowing them to retain the gentle spirit that comes clothed in a new, still unformed and fragile body. And it helps that body adjust to the stimulation of a world full of noises, lights, movement, sharpness, and clamor with curiosity, not fear. Later I learned from many mothers and grandmothers this ancient art of heart and hands that so clearly impacts the bodies, minds, and spirits of the people who receive it.

My first child was born in 1976, and I began massaging him every day. Having taught yoga for several years, I found that a number of its massage techniques and poses were easily incorporated into our daily massage routine—a routine based on my own combination of ancient Indian and modern Swedish methods along with

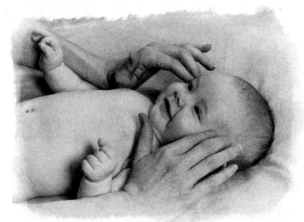

techniques I knew as a yoga instructor. This joyful blend provided my son with a wonderful balance of outgoing and incoming energy, of tension release and stimulation. Additionally, it seemed to relieve the painful gas he had experienced that first month. Gentle yoga-like exercises ended our massage playfully and further helped in toning and relieving his digestive system.

When I massaged my baby with a fully present mind, relaxed body, and open heart, he appeared to relax and was happier for the rest of the day. When I stopped massaging him for two weeks, the change was noticeable. He seemed to carry tension with him and to express more general irritability and fussiness, with painful attacks of colic keeping us up for hours in the night. From that point on I decided that massage would remain a permanent part of our lives—not only as a tool for relaxation and stress relief, but as a key part of our communication with each other.

When my son was seven months old, I decided to develop a curriculum and share my discoveries with other parents. Since then thousands of parents and infants have attended my classes and private instruction. Over the years, they provided me with continuing education and inspiration, for which I am most grateful.

In the years since my early classes, interest in infant massage has grown steadily among parents and professionals alike. I began training instructors, then trained trainers to train instructors. We now have an international nonprofit organization, the first and largest of its kind, for the preservation and dissemination of this ancient practice: the International Association of Infant Massage, with chapters in more than twenty-seven countries. Many hospitals now train nursery staff to use massage and holding techniques with premature and sick babies and offer instruction to parents in an effort to promote bonding and ease babies' discomforts. In addition, the benefits of this simple tradition, intuitively developed and refined in the "laboratories" of thousands of years of human experience, are being recognized day by day in modern scientific research. (I have met with many a joke in this regard, teased gently as a Westerner

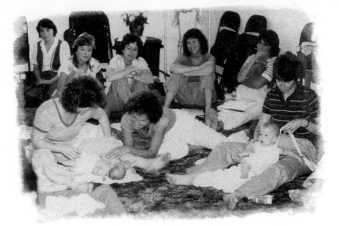

who needs double-blind studies to prove that grass grows if you water it!)

My children are grown now, and the impact of our experience with massage during their infancies has not diminished. The daily massages provided a foundation for physical, emotional, and spiritual harmony and closeness that we all carry with us for life.

I would like to share a letter I received from a mother who learned infant massage from this book when I first began teaching. It is not meant as medical advice; certainly if your baby has medical problems, you should work with your medical professionals and be sure the massage you deliver is appropriate for your baby's needs. I share it with you to show you how profoundly this simple practice can affect a family. I thank the mother who sent me this priceless letter.

Dear Vimala,

I wanted to personally write and thank you for the invaluable contribution you made to my children.

My son was born addicted to a drug that I had been given to stop seizures from toxemia and premature labor. Additionally, I was treated several times with other intravenous drugs. Throughout the pregnancy, repeated physicians scolded me and my husband for continuing the pregnancy. We were assured that our baby would be handicapped, a "vegetable," and so on. We fought hard and well as he survived to thirty-eight weeks gestation, born at a robust eight pounds, fifteen ounces. It was soon obvious that his nervous system was badly affected by the drugs and stress.

He cried endlessly or slept nonstop, missing feedings. If he was startled, his little arms and legs would jut out and shake uncontrollably. The doctors suggested more drugs to calm him. They again asserted that his nervous system (and probably brain) were irreparably harmed. A wonderful neighbor and breastfeeding professional came to our rescue. She taught me your methods of infant massage to calm him and showed me how to swaddle him to prevent jarring his sensitive nervous system. To make a long story a tad bit shorter, he grew to be an inquisitive and absolutely delightful toddler. The shaking subsided, and a brilliant intellect came forth combined with an energy that was tiring to us poor adults. Today, my supposedly "handicapped" child is in college, a National Merit Scholar, a recognized leader, a wonderful volunteer worker, and engaged to be married to a dynamic and equally bright young woman. He was nationally recognized as a teen and was offered more than $375,000 in scholarships. He works with severely handicapped adults and plans on being a physician.

My second son was also the product of a terribly high-risk pregnancy. Drug therapies were a bit more advanced and, with the help of diet, controlled the toxemia. He was born with noted neurological deficits. By the age of five months, we were cautioned that he had begun to show the symptoms of autism. He was highly irritable and, to put it simply, a challenging baby.

I once again drew on my experience with massage. The tension in his little limbs would melt away, and he remained in contact with the world. I kept him close to me, leaving him only with caregivers for short periods of time who were willing to comfort him as needed, to hold him, massage him. Though still plagued with a few problems, he is a very bright and caring sixteen-year-old. He is already doing computer design for toy and software companies.

Without the help of my neighbor who had studied your techniques, I do not believe that either of these young men would be where they are today. I believe that their intellectual, physical, and emotional development is attributable to the comfort they received as infants. How can I ever thank you? Please know that this mother will be in your debt forever.

Sincerely,
A grateful mother

Infant massage can promote the kind of parenting that this attentive mother was able to provide. Its benefits go far beyond the immediate physiological gains. As you massage your baby regularly, you will discover that you develop a bond with your child that will last a lifetime.

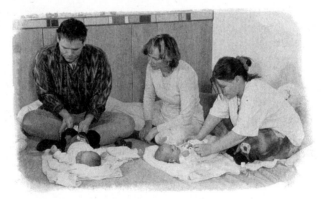

ON CHOOSING THE RIGHT WORD

Like many authors, I have encountered the male-female pronoun problem. When referring to a baby, do I say, "he or she"? Or "he/she"? Or "s/he"? All of these seem clumsy and forced. So to get my own message across as simply as possible, I have chosen to refer to the baby as "he" some of the time, and "she" some of the time—providing balance for all.

Another problem is in reference to the person massaging the baby. I have used "mother" as the primary masseuse in the book both for the sake of convenience and because, in my experience, she is most often principally involved in this care. In addition, massage, as I see it, is a "mothering" activity, whether it is performed by mother or father, brother or sister, grandma or grandpa.

Since it is my sincere hope that fathers may be equally interested and involved, I have included a special section for them. To those fathers who read the book in its entirety and decide to massage their babies, I would simply ask them to change "mother" to "father" in their minds at the appropriate places.

Enough said!

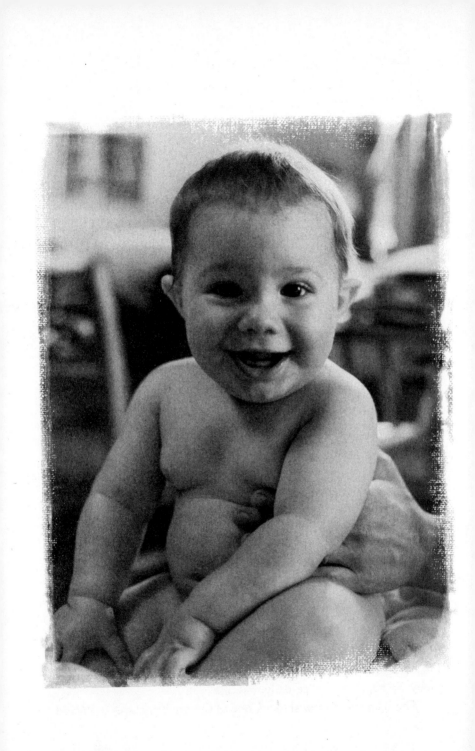

Chapter 1

Why Massage Your Baby?

Being touched and caressed,
Being massaged, is food for the infant.
Food as necessary as minerals,
Vitamins, and proteins.
                    —Dr. Frederick Leboyer

AN AGE-OLD TRADITION

A YOUNG MOTHER gently cradles her baby in her lap as the afternoon sun breaks through cracks in the wooden door. For the second time that day, she carefully removes the tiny cap and begins to unwrap the swaddling bands of soft white linen and wool.

Freed from his snug encasement, the baby kicks and waves his little arms, listening to the now-familiar swish-swish of the warm oil in his mother's hands, and the comforting sound of her balmy lullaby. So begins his twice-daily massage.

The scene is in a Jewish *shtetl*, one of the small enclaves in Poland in the early nineteenth century, but we could be anywhere in the world, in any century, for it is a familiar tableau of motherhood in every culture throughout the ages.

From the Eskimos of the Canadian Arctic to the Ganda of East Africa; from South India to Northern Ireland; in Russia, China, Sweden, and South America; in South Sea island huts and modern American homes, babies are lovingly massaged, caressed, and crooned to every day. Mothers all over the world know their babies need to be held, carried, rocked, and touched. The gentle art of infant massage has been part of baby caregiving traditions passed from parent to child for generations. Asked why, each culture would provide different answers. Most would simply say, "It is our custom."

Many of the family customs of our ancestors, turned aside in the early twentieth century in the interest of "progress," are returning to our lives as modern science rediscovers their importance and their contribution to our infants' well-being and that of whole communities. Cross-cultural studies have demonstrated that in societies where infants are held, massaged, rocked, breastfed, and carried, adults are less aggressive and violent, more cooperative and compassionate. Our great-grandmothers would stand up and utter a great "I told you so!" were they to observe our "new" discoveries in infant care.

CAN BABIES BE SPOILED WITH LOVE?

Research can help us understand why these traditional practices are so important. Knowing why, we will be less quick to cast adrift customs that can deeply enrich our lives. Nearly every new parent hears the admonition "Don't spoil the baby!" at one time or another in the early months of parenting. Our concern about raising "spoiled" children comes from an earlier time when behaviorists, after discovering behavioral conditioning, thought that we could condition our babies to behave like little adults by ignoring their cries and not offering too much affection.

That approach has become popular again. (Fads swing like a

pendulum from one extreme to another, and parenting advice of course is not immune to this phenomenon.) In the late 1990s, a popular baby care program advised parents to put babies on rigid schedules, allow them to cry alone, and punish them for behavior that was not convenient for parents. The leaders of this movement also managed to convince parents that they damaged their infant's metabolism by breastfeeding on demand (all research to the contrary) and created spoiled, selfish children if parents responded to their needs and comforted them when they cried. Parents were admonished never to allow their infants to sleep with them, for they could easily kill them (again, all research to the contrary). This represented a swing away from the natural parenting practices that had gained momentum in the 1970s and achieved recognition from pediatricians as healthy and normal by the 1990s.

Proof abounds that babies who are neglected and punished suffer bonding breaks and, without intervention, often grow up to be troubled if not antisocial or sociopathic individuals. In my more than twenty years of working with parents to bond more deeply with their infants, respect them, learn their nonverbal "language," and respond to them with love, I have received countless letters from parents saying infant massage changed their entire life as a family, and their children turned out to be lively, creative, inquisitive, secure, intelligent, social, loving, humanitarian human beings. Authoritarian advisers neglect to mention that parents all over the world have naturally responded with love to their babies, breastfed on demand, slept in "family beds," and carried infants in various types of slings—for millennia—and that if you read the biographies of terrorists, serial killers, and cruel dictators, you will invariably find neglected or authoritarian childhoods.

Infant massage, as it is shared in this book, is not a fad. It is an ancient art that connects you deeply with the person who is your baby, and it helps you to understand your baby's particular nonverbal language and respond with love and respectful listening. It empowers you as a parent, for it gives you the means by which you become an expert on your own child and therefore can respond according to your baby's unique needs. Rather than growing up selfish and demanding (though all kids go through such stages), a child whose voice is heard, whose heart is full, and who is enveloped in love overflows with that love and naturally, unselfconsciously gives of himself to others. He learns what healthy, respectful touch is by being touched that way. He learns self-discipline by watching his parents and imitating them. He has little to rebel against because there is no festering resentment of parents' authoritarian or autocratic, unpredictable rules and punishments. The deep emotional bonds formed in infancy lay a foundation for a lifetime of trust, courage, dependability, faith, and love.

Infant massage is not just for parents who embrace a certain lifestyle. Whether your baby sleeps with you or in her own room, is breast- or bottle-fed, is weaned early or late—all these decisions are up to you. Massaging your baby simply communicates love, releases tension, and helps you better understand your baby's needs. The fact that it is fun is a wonderful added benefit!

After more than fifty years of intensive research, it has become obvious that, as with fruit, neglect rather than attention spoils a child. "I'd gotten so much pressure about spoiling the baby, even before she was born," says Judith, mother of three-year-old Kelsey. "But I felt dif-

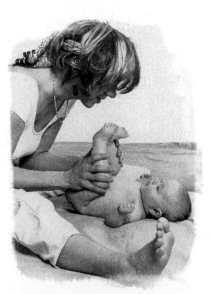

ferently inside. The information about the benefits of infant massage gave me permission to be the kind of mother I want to be and the research to back me up when I am contradicted." When we know why our caress is so important to our babies, we are more likely to follow our intuition, to relax, and to give way to our natural inclinations.

Both for babies and parents, the benefits of infant massage are more far-reaching than they may at first seem. For an infant, massage is much more than a luxurious, sensual experience or a type of physical therapy. It is a tool for maintaining a child's health and well-being on many levels. It helps parents feel secure in their ability to do something positive for—and get a positive response from—this squealing bit of newborn humanity suddenly and urgently put in their charge.

THE BENEFITS OF SKIN STIMULATION

Skin sensitivity is one of the earliest developed and most fundamental functions of the body. Stimulation of the skin is, in fact, essential for adequate organic and psychological development, both for animals and for human beings. When asked what he thought of infant massage, anthropologist Ashley Montagu commented, "People don't realize that communication for a baby, the first communications it receives and the first language of its development, is through the skin. If only most people had realized this they would have all along given babies the kind of skin stimulation they require."

You may wonder why I started out talking about babies and now switch to animals. It is because scientists have discovered behaviors and responses in animals that often parallel those of our own young. And these parallels are truly fascinating!

Behaviorally, mammals tend to fall into the "cache" or "carry" type. The caching species leave their young for long periods while the mother gathers food. The infants must remain silent for long periods of time so as not to attract predators; therefore they do not cry. For the same reason, they do not urinate unless stimulated by the mother. In addition, the young have internal mechanisms that control their body temperature. The mother's milk is extremely high in protein and fat, and the infants suckle at a very fast rate.

In contrast, the carrying species maintain continuous contact with their infants and feed often. The babies suckle slowly, they urinate often, they cry when distressed or out of contact with the parent, and they need the parent to keep them warm. The mother's milk content is low in protein and fat, so infants need to suckle often. Humans are designed like the carrying species; in fact, human milk is identical in protein and fat content to that of the anthropoid apes, a carrying species. Our infants need to be in close physical contact with us as much as possible.

Harry Harlow's famous monkey experiments were the first to show that for infants, contact comfort is even more important than food. Infant monkeys, given the choice of a wire mother figure with food or a soft, terrycloth figure without food, chose the terrycloth mother figure. Human infants with failure-to-thrive syndrome exhibit the same type of behavior; though given all the food they need, they continue to deteriorate without intervention that involves emotional nurturing, contact comfort, and care.

Physically, massage acts in much the same way in humans as licking does in animals. Animals lick their young and maintain close skin contact. Animals that are not licked, caressed, or permitted to cling in infancy grow up scrawny and more vulnerable to stress. They tend to fight with one another and to abuse and neglect their own young. Licking serves to stimulate the physiological systems and to bond the young with the mother. A mother cat spends over fifty percent of her time licking her babies—and you will never see a colicky kitten! In fact, without the kind of stimulation that helps their gastrointestinal system begin to function properly, newborn kittens die.

In one study, rats with their thyroid and parathyroid (endocrine glands that regulate the immune system) removed responded remarkably to massage. In the experimental group, the rats were gently massaged and spoken to several times a day. They were relaxed and yielding and not easily frightened, and their nervous systems remained stable. The control group rats, which did not receive this type of care, were nervous, fearful, irritable, and enraged: they died within forty-eight hours. Another study with rats showed a higher immunity to disease, faster weight gain, and better neurological development among those that had been gently stroked in infancy.

Moving up the animal scale, dogs, horses, cows, dolphins, and many other animals have also shown remarkable differences when lovingly handled in infancy. Gentle touching and stroking improved the function of virtually all the sustaining systems (respiratory, circulatory, digestive, eliminative, nervous, and endocrine) and changed behavior patterns drastically, reducing fear and excitement thresholds and in-

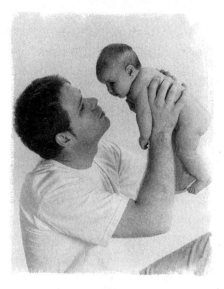

creasing gentleness, friendliness, and fearlessness. In his book *Touching*, Ashley Montagu writes: "the more we learn about the effects of cutaneous [skin] stimulation, the more pervasively significant for healthy development do we find it to be."

In nearly every bird and mammal studied, close physical contact has been found to be essential both to the infant's healthy survival and to the mother's ability to nurture. In the previously mentioned studies with rats, if pregnant females were restrained from licking themselves (a form of self-massage), their mothering activities were substantially diminished. Additionally, when pregnant female animals were gently stroked every day, their offspring showed higher weight gain and reduced excitability, and the mothers showed greater interest in their offspring, with a more abundant and richer milk supply.

Evidence supports the same conclusions for humans. Studies with premature babies using techniques similar to those taught in this book have demonstrated that daily massage is of tremendous benefit. Research projects at the University of Miami Medical Center, headed up by the Touch Research Institute's founder, Dr. Tiffany Field, have shown remarkable results. In one study, twenty premature babies were massaged three times a day for fifteen minutes each. They averaged forty-seven percent greater weight gain per day, were more active and alert, and showed more mature neurological development than infants who did not receive massage. In addition, their hospital stay averaged six days less.

Dallas psychologist Ruth Rice conducted a study with thirty premature babies after they had left the hospital. She divided them into two groups. The mothers in the control group were instructed in usual newborn care, while those in the experimental group were taught a daily massage and rocking regime. At four months of age, the babies who had been massaged were ahead in both neurological development and weight gain.

The natural sensory stimulation of massage speeds myelination of the brain and the nervous system. The myelin sheath is a fatty covering around each nerve, like insulation around electrical wire. It protects the nervous system and speeds the transmission of impulses from the brain to the rest of the body. The process of coating the nerves is not complete at birth, but skin stimulation speeds the process, thus enhancing rapid neural-cell firing and improving brain-body communication.

In 1978 transcutaneous oxygen monitoring was developed, which enabled physicians to measure oxygen tension in the body through an electrode on the skin. It was discovered that hospitalized infants experienced tremendous upheavals in oxygen levels when subjected to stress. Massage and Touch Relaxation (see Chapter 5) have been found to mitigate these fluctuations, and these methods are being used in hospitals routinely now to help infants maintain a steady state through the stresses of diaper changes, heel sticks, and other intrusions.

New research demonstrates similar results every day, confirming what age-old tradition has told us: infants need loving touch. Lawrence Schachner, M.D., a professor at the department of dermatology and cutaneous surgery at the University of Miami School of Medicine, advises that touch can benefit babies with skin disorders such as eczema. "It may furthermore improve parent-baby interaction," he says. Dr. Tiffany Field concurs: "Our research suggests that touch is as important to infants and children as eating and sleeping." She notes that loving touch triggers physiological changes that help infants grow and develop, stimulating nerves in the brain that facilitate food absorption and lowering stress hormone levels, resulting in improved immune system functioning. A report by the Families and Work Institute states that during the first three years of life, the vast majority of connections between brain cells are formed. They conclude that loving interaction such as massage can directly affect a child's emotional development and ability to handle stress as an adult.

Loving skin contact and massage benefits mothers and fathers as well. Mothers who have meaningful skin contact during pregnancy and labor tend to have easier labors and are more responsive to their infants. In addition, research has shown that mothers whose pregnancies were filled with chronic stress often have babies who cry more and for longer periods than those whose pregnancies were peaceful and supported.

Fathers who make the effort to bond with their infants by giving the mother loving massages, talking to the baby, feeling its movements in their partner's belly, attending classes with their partner, and reading up on infant development and psychology, tend to be more attentive and accomplished fathers. By regularly massaging your baby (and getting some loving massages yourself during pregnancy), you set up a cycle of healthy responses that improve your mothering skills day by day and enhance your baby's well-being, disposition, and the relationship among all three of you.

STRESS AND RELAXATION

In our great-grandmothers' day, when a baby developed a fever, the outcome was uncertain. Each century's children have been plagued with some debilitating disease. Though many contagions have been eliminated through improved environmental conditions and medicine, our century is characterized by a more subtle and insidious malady—stress.

Stress can begin to affect a baby even before he is born. The levels of stress hormones that are constantly present in a woman's bloodstream directly affect her unborn infant, crossing the placenta to enter his own bloodstream. Studies have shown that prolonged tension and anxiety can hamper a pregnant woman's ability to absorb nourishment. Her baby may be of low birth weight, hyperactive, and irritable.

If we understand that our experiences and reactions influence our own biochemistry by sending life-enhancing or fear-producing chemicals throughout our bodies, it is not difficult to understand that these chemicals are also sent through our unborn baby's body. Her cells receive this "information" and program her structure accordingly. Thus, even before birth, a baby can unconsciously perceive the world as a place of anxiety and stress, to fight or be victimized by, or a place of safety and love, to enjoy and fully experience. This is not to say all is lost if life circumstances are less than perfect. Infant massage is one tool we have to help reshape our child's interpretations of the world, to release her pain, grief, and fear, and to open her up to love and joy. As we evolve to be more conscious beings, we understand more deeply how important our mind states are, both to our own health and longevity and to our children's health, longevity, intelligence, and ability to experience and give love and joy.

Babies born centuries ago in more primitive cultures had the advantage of extended families, natural environments, and relatively little change. Our children, born into a rapidly advancing technological world, must effectively handle stress if they are to survive and prosper. Thus we must give them every opportunity, from conception on, to learn positive, adaptive responses to stress and to believe in their own power and adaptability.

We certainly cannot eliminate stress, nor would we wish to, for in the proper doses it is an essential component in the growth of intelligence. Let's see how this works. In times of stress, the pituitary gland produces a hormone called ACTH (adrenocorticotropic hormone), which activates the adrenal steroids, organizing the body and brain to deal with an unknown or unpredictable emergency. In experiments with laboratory animals, this hormone has been found to stimulate the production of many new proteins in the liver and brain—proteins that are instrumental in both learning and memory. On being given ACTH, the animals' brains grow millions of new connecting links between the neurons (thinking cells). These links enable the brain to process information.

The stress of meeting unknown situations and converting them into what is known and predictable is essential for our babies' brain development. But stress is only part of the cycle that enhances learning. Without its equally important opposite—relaxation—stress can lead to overstimulation, exhaustion, and shock. When stress piles upon stress without the relief of an equal portion of relaxation, the body begins to shut out all sensory intake and the learning process is completely blocked. As neuroscientist Bruce Lipton described, between the two choices—protection-related or growth-promoting—protection-related biological behaviors kick in, thus preventing growth or learning.

How does this apply to infant massage? First, massage is one way we can provide our children with relaxing, joyful experiences. Through the use of conditioned response techniques similar to those developed for childbirth by Lamaze and others, we can teach our babies how to relax their bodies in response to stress. The ability to relax consciously is a tremendous advantage in coping with the pressures of growing up in modern society. If acquired early in life, the relaxation response can become as much a part of our children's natural system as the antibodies that protect them from disease.

Stress is a natural part of an infant's life, but often our babies are not able to benefit from it as much as they could. Our fast-paced society overloads them with input, but it is unacceptable for them to cry to release tension. This double bind leads to many frustrated babies with a lot of pent-up tension and anxiety.

Massage helps babies practice handling input and responding to it with relaxation. Watch an experienced mother massaging her baby. You will see both stress and relaxation in the rhythmic strokes and in the baby's reactions. The infant experiences all kinds of new sensations, feelings, odors, sounds, and sights. The rumbles of his tummy, the warm sensation of increased circulation, the movement of air on his bare skin—all are mildly stressful to him. The pleasant tone of his mother's voice, her smile and her touch are relaxing and relieve the discomfort of encountering these new sensations. She reassures him that the world outside the womb is, as Dr. Frederick Leboyer says, "still alive, and warm, and beating, and friendly."

A daily massage raises an infant's stimulation threshold. Babies who have difficulty handling stimulation gradually build tolerance. High-need babies begin to learn to regulate the manner in which they respond to stressful experiences, which reduces the level of tension they develop throughout the day. Colicky babies are calmed and able to relax their bodies so that tension doesn't escalate their discomfort. A regular massage provides our babies with an early stress management program that will be valuable to them in years to come.

INTO ADULTHOOD

Psychologists study the types of attachments we form in our infancy as predictors of the types of relationships we will have as adults. People whose infancy was secure, who were held and listened to, who had good eye contact with their parents, and who were generally cherished tend to have healthier relationships with others. Getting close to others is easy, and they have no problem with interdependency (the ability to depend on and be depended on, appropriately). They have happy, trusting relationships; their romances last the longest and end in divorce the least often of groups studied. On the other hand, babies whose attachment bonds are insecure or anxious are later less sympathetic to others and less effective in getting support and help from other people. Their relationships lack trust and intimacy; jealousy, commitment problems, and fears undermine friendships as well as marriages. People whose bonds are constantly broken in infancy have a much greater risk of becoming sociopathic criminals in their adulthood, unless they receive serious intervention at an early age.

The bonds of trust and love, the lessons of compassion, warmth, openness, and respect that are inherent in the massage routine will be carried by your child into adulthood. Especially if your parenting practices reflect the same values of infant massage, your child will be more likely to respond to others with empathy and warmth, to respond to social problems with compassion and altruism, and to experience life as a joyful adventure in which he has the opportunity to love and be loved—to help others and extend himself in genuine service to humanity.

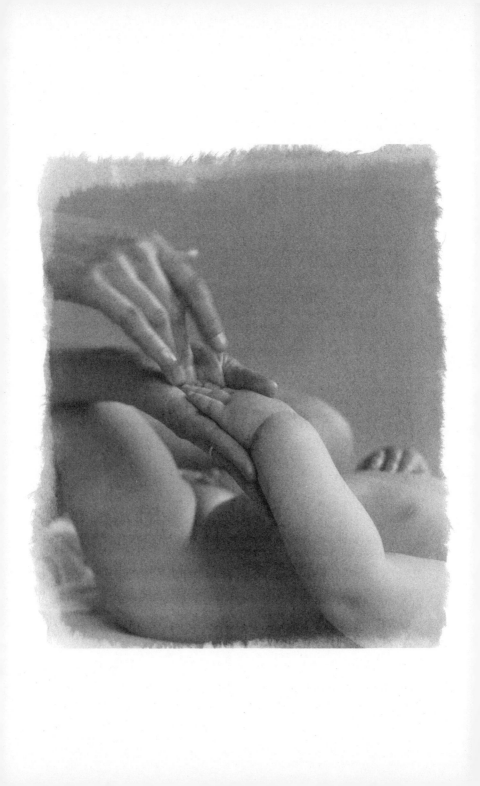

Chapter 2

Your Baby's
Sensory World

🌿

Two little eyes to look around,
Two little ears to hear a sound,
One little nose to smell what's sweet,
One little mouth that likes to eat.
   —Traditional nursery rhyme

AN INFANT'S SENSES develop in sequence: first the proximity senses (those that need the nearness of some object to operate effectively), and then the distance senses (those that help the baby perceive things that are farther away). Of the proximity senses, the first and most important is touch.

TOUCH AND MOVEMENT

The sense of touch has been detected in human embryos less than eight weeks old. Though the baby is less than an inch long and has no eyes or ears, her skin sensitivity is already highly developed.

Nature begins the baby's massage long before she is born. First she rocks and floats, then slowly her world surrounds her ever more closely. The gentle caress of the womb becomes stronger, gradually becoming the contractions that rhythmically squeeze and push, providing massive stimulation to the infant's skin and organ systems.

Infants are accustomed to the tactile stimulation of constant movement, and they need the reestablishment of those rhythms after birth. In two studies, mothers in one group were asked to carry their infants not only during feeding or crying but for extra periods of time each day, in a soft front pack. These infants were compared with infants who were held and carried normally. At six weeks, the infants who received the extra touching and movement cried half as much as the others. Today Kangaroo Care is a common practice in hospital nurseries because of its beneficial effects on premature infants' physiological, social-emotional, and psychological health. Similarly, premature babies often receive massage as part of their care, now that Dr. Tiffany Field's studies have proven its remarkable impact on growth and development.

TASTE AND SMELL

Other proximity senses are taste and smell, both of which are connected with touch and are significant to the newborn. A baby only five days old can differentiate her mother's smell and the taste of her milk from that of another mother. Infants, too, have special "chemical signatures" that their mothers are able to detect. Research shows that many mothers can pick out their infants' garments by scent alone after only two hours of exposure to their newborns.

SIGHT AND HEARING

The distance senses—sight and hearing—can be very important to a baby's emotional attachment to his mother, an attachment that is essential to the development of a healthy parent-baby relationship. But the baby with a hearing and/or visual impairment will not suffer from lack of this bond if he has conscientious parents; the sense of touch and its impact upon maternal attachment is equally powerful. In fact, touch may be more dynamic, because it is the most significant and highly developed sense.

Even before birth, your baby can see. Before you know you are pregnant, the baby's optic nerve (the structure that transmits signals from the eye to the brain) has been formed. By six to seven months gestation, the baby's brain responds to light, and she can open and close her eyes, look up, down, and sideways. Your newborn is programmed to see you. Her eyes focus quite clearly at around seven to twelve inches—the distance at which your arms hold her comfortably. She is especially attracted to the high-contrast, bull's-eye shapes of your eyes and nipples; this attraction enhances bonding through eye and skin contact and thus ensures her survival. In addition, the stimulation of gazing at these objects may enhance nerve myelination and physiological development.

A mother's instinctive use of a high-pitched voice fits in beautifully with her baby's natural attraction to higher-frequency speech. The association between auditory and visual centers is fully established as early as two weeks of age. Your baby likes to look at you and hear your voice. In one experiment, babies were given four configurations of speech and sight from which to choose: the mother speaking normally, a stranger speaking normally, a stranger speaking with the mother's voice, and the mother speaking with a stranger's voice. The mother speaking normally was bliss. The babies looked less at a stranger speaking normally. But, the mother-stranger mixes were intolerable, and the infants reacted with loud crying whenever they were presented to them. In another experiment, newborn infants were

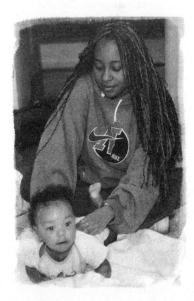

fitted with headphones through which they heard a voice telling a story. Whenever they sucked rapidly on a pacifier, they would hear their mothers' voices; otherwise a stranger told the story. The infants learned how to cause their mothers' voices to tell the story, and they preferred their mothers' voices to any other.

The beginnings of language learning can be seen in a baby's movement of her body in rhythm and synchrony with her mother's speech patterns, intonations, and pauses. Computer studies analyzing movies of mothers and babies have revealed that each infant has a unique repertoire of body movements that synchronize with speech—a bodily response for every speech pattern. As the child grows older, these movements become microkinetic—discernible only through sophisticated instrumentation. At first the baby displays constant reflex movements, followed by the development of vocalization, then inflections, emotional content, and babbling. Finally words come, and ultimately these words have meaning of their own, no longer needing the reflex motor movements. But even a preschool child will move her foot when you ask her to say the word *foot*. There is still a trace of the parent's voice, internalized, saying "foot" as the infant body responds. The sounds a parent makes, including "parentese" or baby talk and rhythmic songs and rhymes, appeal directly to the baby's right brain hemisphere, which is more highly developed at this stage.

The baby has been hearing his parents' voices from the time hearing developed in the womb, and the rhythms of speech even before that, through the reverberations of sounds that travel through the mother's bones. It is now believed that babies can begin to decipher language as early as six weeks of age. Other studies have shown that babies can differentiate different types of sentence structure and certain words that seem to go together, such as *the* before *dog*.

In 1997 studies by University of Washington neuroscientist Patricia Kuhl showed that parents unconsciously exaggerate vowel sounds, which help babies develop a mastery of the phonetics of speech. For example, the word *bead*, she says, could easily be confused with *bed* or *bid*. But parents speak to their babies in "baby talk," saying, "Look at Mommy's beeeeeeds," in a high-pitched, singsong manner that stresses and exaggerates the vowels. Parents naturally provide the distinctions between vowel sounds that help their children learn to speak and, later, to read.

Kuhl had found that six-month-olds categorize vowel sounds that are meaningful in their native language. She found parents' exaggeration of vowel sounds to be universal, in any language she studied. So it seems we are "programmed" to provide the auditory information that our babies need in order to begin to understand and speak their native tongue. Later, when we begin doing infant massage, you will find that certain strokes can have rhymes or sounds associated with them, which accomplishes this same goal. While doing the stroke called "I Love You" on the baby's tummy, I encourage parents to elongate the vowels in a high-pitched voice. In every infant massage class I have taught or observed, the babies immediately attune to and are delighted with this particular stroke. Often, if some of the babies are fussing, all the parents in the room may simultaneously do the "I Love You" stroke, saying the words aloud with the sounds elongated. The fussing stops, and all the babies giggle and smile with rapt attention as the stroke is repeated. This stroke is the one most often requested by toddlers as well, who like to repeat the sounds with their parents as the stroke is done.

"INFANT STIM"

While no one argues that infants are drawn naturally to the types of stimulation they need for healthy development, researchers do disagree about the value of artificially stimulating an infant's senses. Advocates of early stimulation say that looking at stark black-and-white images (such as mobiles made of black-and-white bull's-eyes, checkerboards, and stripes), listening to recordings, including recordings of "white noise" (monotonous sounds such as vacuum cleaners and car engines), and other sensory stimuli may speed an infant's development and increase his intelligence, help an infant sleep, or soothe his colic.

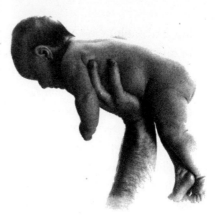

Henry Williams, M.D., a widely respected physician and former chairman of the Anthroposophical Society's Fellowship of Physicians, proposes that infants have come from a place of soft contours and hazy colors, and that it is reasonable that they be introduced gradually to the hard edges of the world in which they have just arrived. "We want to bring them gently into life on this plane of existence," he says, "to make it a quiet, careful transition with soft music, modified contours, and muted colors, slowly introducing them to these edges of things that can be so fascinating because they are new. There is no rush about it."

Our great concern about our children's ability to compete on intelligence tests can drive us to accept programs that may or may not be valuable and that may in fact be detrimental to a child's long-range emotional and spiritual development. Especially makers of products for babies imply that our children will not be able to compete for money and status in an increasingly competitive environment unless they are weaned to certain objects and ways of processing information as early as possible. Attaching the infant to material objects as "sensory stimulators" certainly benefits the companies that produce the products and the experts who promote them. At the same time, parents, who receive little or no cultural support for their role, are often relieved of stress and guilt by these mechanical interventions. I am concerned about our slowly deteriorating intuitive abilities and confidence in ourselves. We may one day come to believe that material objects are actually better stimulators, more competent soothers, and more efficient brain-developers than we are, and that without these products our babies will be deprived. Instead of providing emotional nurturing, spiritual teaching, and exploration of the living world, we work harder and harder to provide our infants with the "necessary" objects of stimulation.

As researchers become more interested in the incredible array of benefits that massage can bring to infants, their interest has not gone unnoticed by profit seekers. Many years ago I joked that if we wanted to make a lot of money, we could make a "baby massage device" that could be turned on and applied to the baby. The only problem would be that all of the benefits of infant massage would be forfeited. To my immense shock and dismay, a company has actually made a "baby massager," similar to the shiatsu massage devices so popular in malls (which usually end up in the closet, because nothing can ease tension like human touch). Many unknowing parents will buy it, thinking it will benefit their babies. But these, too, will end up in the closet, as parents realize that nothing can replace their loving hands.

Developmental psychologists today agree that infants are natural learners and will extract from a warm, loving environment whatever information they need. The basic security provided by a strong parent-infant bond enables babies to reach out to their world and to develop to their full capacity physically, mentally, and spiritually. Infant massage provides a wealth of fascinating sensory experiences. Your eyes, your hairline, your smile, your scent, and the sound of your voice telling a story or singing a lullaby provide not only the interesting contrast your baby looks for but also warm, loving feedback. It not only speeds the myelination of her nerves, it lets her know she has come into a living, breathing world. There is no sweeter music than the sound of a mother singing; there will never be a toy that can tell a story the way a real, live daddy can. No one can invent a substitute for a parent's loving touch. No vestibular stimulation device can compare with being rocked and carried in loving arms. And as for white noise, nothing can surpass the sounds of breath and heart in synchrony.

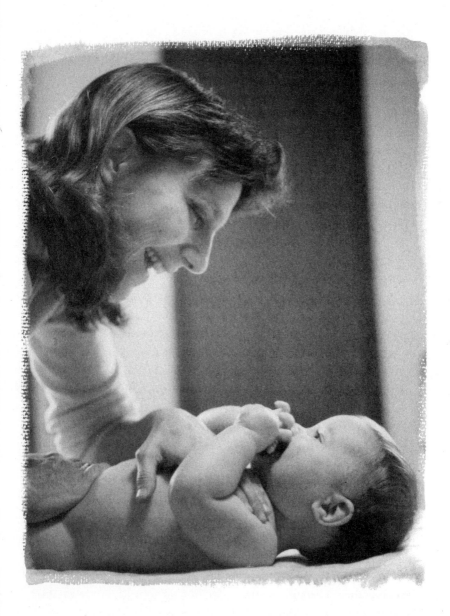

Chapter 3

Bonding, Attachment, and Infant Massage

Baby, I lie and gaze on thee
All other things forgot—
In dreams the things of earth pass by
But awake I heed them not.
I hear thy soft breath come and go,
Thy breath so lately given,
And watch the blue unconscious eyes
Whose light is pure from heaven.
　　　　—Anonymous, 1860

THE IMPORTANCE OF BONDING AND ATTACHMENT TO YOUR BABY

BONDING IS A BASIC phenomenon that occurs throughout the universe. In terms of physics, it is established within the energy field from which particles arise. Two particles of energy brought into proximity spin and polarize identically, even when separated. Two living cells of a human heart brought into proximity begin to beat together. Throughout the animal kingdom and in human life as well, affectionate and tactile bonds between mother and young ensure healthy interaction and development for time to come. Proximity between parent and infant, via sensory experiences and loving interactions, brings them into an important synchrony with each other.

Animal researchers discovered imprinting long ago, when ethologist Konrad Lorenz showed that ducklings were biologically programmed to follow and bond with the first moving object they saw. Meanwhile, Harry Harlow and his associates studied monkeys and goats and found critical bonding times and elements that were important not only for the infant's physical survival but for what we might call emotional health as well. Monkeys would abuse their infants if their own bonds as infants had been disturbed.

In animals, the crucial period for bonding is usually a matter of minutes or hours after birth. The mother bonds with her infant through licking and touching, a type of massage, which in turn helps the infant to adjust physically to life outside the womb. If mother and infant are separated during this time and are subsequently reunited, the mother will often reject or neglect her young. As a result, the newborn may die for lack of the mother's stimulation, even if fed by other means.

In studies paralleling animal research, doctors John Kennell and Marshall Klaus, among others, have revealed that there is also a sensitive period for bonding in humans. But the critical period seems less rigidly defined and may continue for months, even years, after childbirth. Another word often used in connection with bonding is *attachment*. While bonding is specific to birth and our connection with the animal kingdom, attachment happens over time and can occur between any two beings. Frank Bolton in his book *When Bonding Fails* describes bonding as a one-directional process that begins in the biological mother during pregnancy and continues through birth and the first days of her baby's life. Conversely, attachment is an interaction between parents and children, biological or not, that develops during the first year they are together and is reinforced throughout life. He describes it as the feeling that the other is "irreplaceable."

Often these two terms are used interchangeably, because in humans the bonding period is so loosely defined as to merge into the attachment process. Kennell and Klaus define bonding as "a unique relationship between two people that is specific and endures through time." That definition could also apply to the word *attachment*. In this book, I am using these terms interchangeably, as we are not conforming here to strict research or medically oriented language. Rather, we use these concepts in our everyday speech to imply the love that develops between parent and child, whether the child be a birth-parent's newborn or an adopted baby or toddler. Bonding and attachment, as we use them, are the whole continuum of closeness that happens over time and that can be augmented by the practice of infant massage.

Kennell and Klaus cited cuddling, kissing, and prolonged gazing as indicators of a developing bond. Dramatic evidence in their studies and others correlates the lack of early bonding and attachment with later abuse, neglect, and failure to thrive. Mothers who are separated from their babies during the newborn period are often more hesitant to learn and unskilled in basic mothering tasks. Even very short separations sometimes adversely affect the relationship between mothers and infants.

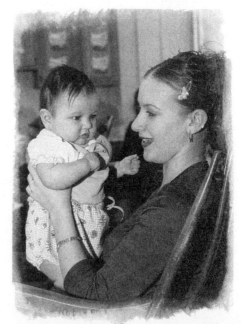

Experts in many fields are becoming increasingly alarmed at what has been termed the "bonding crisis" in Western countries. Long before the outbreak of violence among children in the United States, Dr. Ken Magid, psychologist and author of *High Risk: Children Without a Conscience*, pointed to what he called a "profound demographic revolution" that is changing the course of history. "Working mothers—and the possibility that their children are suffering bonding breaks—are simply not being given enough attention," he said. In 1988, in a chilling foretelling of events to come, he cited the stresses of two-income families, single parents struggling to survive, an achievement-addicted society, poorly run and understaffed day care, little or no parental leave in the job market, poorly handled adoptions, and inadequate child custody divorce arrangements as high-risk factors for our newest generations of infants. Unattached and anxiously attached infants can grow up to exhibit a range of disorders from difficulty in forming and maintaining relationships at one end of the scale all the way to sociopathic criminal behavior at the other. *Anxiously attached* means that a baby is not consistently responded to with love by her caregivers, so the baby cannot relax and depend on her needs being met and the world being a good and friendly place to be. Such children are fearful of the world and have a difficult time trusting and opening up to others, and they often have buried anger that can come out inappropriately later in life. Solid, loving attachments are hard for them to make because as anxiously attached babies, they did not learn how to trust.

Unlike the clinging monkey, the human infant has no physical means of initiating contact with his mother and thus getting his needs fulfilled. His life depends upon the strength of his parent's emotional attachment to him. Where there is early and extended mother-baby contact, studies show impressively positive results. Mothers who bonded with their babies in the first hours and days of life later showed greater closeness to their infants, exhibited much more soothing behavior, maintained more eye contact, and touched their babies more often. Early contact mothers were more successful in breastfeeding and spent more time looking at their infants during feeding, and their babies' weight gain was greater. At age three, these children had significantly higher IQ scores on the Stanford-Binet test than children who had been separated from their mothers.

INFANT DAY CARE

Experts who have studied the effects of day care on babies under one year of age sounded the alarm as early as 1985 when many studies began to support the conclusion that poor quality day care, poor quality home care, and too-early day care can cause long-term stresses and possible damage to important parent-infant bonds.

Many years later we are alarmed at the number of children who have little or no conscience about using violence as a way to gain status, peer acceptance, and relief from fears and frustrations. Though many factors contribute to this phenomenon including the assault of inappropriate media, more tolerance for violence in our culture as a whole, the disintegration of extended family bonds, and the financial pressures that put unreasonable strain on every family, some experts suggest that breaks in the attachment process can go deep into an infant's psychology, engendering rage that finally expresses itself by hurting another being. Separation from the primary parent too early in life can threaten bonds and wreak havoc on the child's later life and family harmony. Children whose bonding has been anxious or inadequate or whose family is unable to exert influence and boundaries on behavior often grow up with serious psychosocial problems that are difficult to address and heal.

Many new parents have little choice with regard to their contribution to the family income, making day care a significant issue for every new family. So the information here is not meant to engender guilt in working parents. It is not day care versus stay-at-home-parenting that is important to evaluate, though that is a decision to be made carefully. I believe the most important aspect of this subject is the quality of care the baby receives, regardless of who delivers it, and the quality of the environment at home when the baby returns. That said, I still believe that parents are a young infant's best caregivers because this is the time when the most important bonds of attachment form, which impact a baby's psychology and behavior, and thus the way she is responded to by peers and culture, for life.

Magid emphasizes the dangers of too-early day care in *High Risk*. "After reviewing all the literature, it is my opinion that no child should be left for any significant period of time during the first year of life," he says. "Parents of small infants must proceed with extreme caution when they are considering turning care of their baby over to someone else, whether it be a babysitter or relative. These are the most important moments of your baby's life."

In research done by the National Institute on Child Health and Development in 1996, 1,300 families were followed as the children grew from infancy to age seven; they were observed both in day-care settings and at home. The study found that infants in low-quality day care or infants who had several different caregivers in day care were more likely to develop anxious or insecure attach-

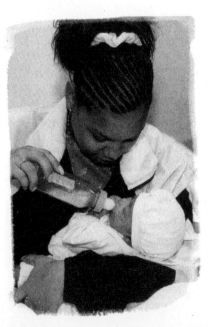

ments if their mothers were also unresponsive to their needs. So it is not necessarily the amount of time an infant is in day care, but the quality of interaction in the family, the quality of environment in the day care, and the quality of interaction with day-care providers (preferably as few as possible) that affects whether an infant can develop healthy bonds.

Studies also show that high-quality day care can prevent the drop in IQ that happens between twelve and thirty months of age in babies kept in home-reared, low-income environments. It seems that whether an infant is in day care is not the most important issue. A stressful environment in which an infant is not given the love, affection, and relaxed attention he needs seems to be the highest risk factor for developing an attachment disorder. Thus, even if a parent stays home to care for a baby, if the loss of income and self-esteem puts the parent under undue stress, this in itself will affect the baby adversely, more so than if the baby was in a high-quality day-care situation with one or two consistent, loving caregivers, and the parents were happy at home and could provide the baby with love, affection, play, and focused attention outside of work.

Parents who simply cannot take time off from work to care for their newborn infants get little help from our culture in providing substitute care that is of acceptable quality. They must suffer the anguish of separation from their infants, the feelings of guilt that result, and worries about the adequacy of the care they have chosen. Often these feelings in themselves serve to distance parents from their infants and further deteriorate bonds that should be strengthened.

A daily massage can be of tremendous help in maintaining and strengthening affectionate bonds between parents and an infant in day care. Taking a half hour for reconnecting through massage after work can help a parent refocus on home life and help an infant to feel secure and supported.

"Our baby loves his massage and typically smiles and coos throughout," says Barbara, mother of six-month-old John. "Since both my husband and I work outside the home, the massage is a way to tune out work and reconnect with John and each other after a stressful day. We are convinced that our baby is happy and relaxed because of the time we spend massaging him."

Other working parents find that their infants often spend part of the massage time fussing. One mother told me she thought her baby liked the day-care provider more than her, because he always cried hard the first hour or so at home and fussed through the first part of his massage, whereas he seemed very happy in day care. Often she just stopped massaging him and let him cry himself to sleep, frustrated and feeling inadequate as a parent. Her view of the situation changed when I suggested that his crying indicated just the opposite: he saved his expression of stress until he was with her, the most safe environment in which he could release pent-up tension from all the day's stimulation. Considering his crying this way, she could help him release his stress by empathizing with him through her voice and body language, and continuing the massage using holding techniques and stopping for comfort breaks. Within a few weeks, her baby cried less and less. Eventually, they bonded closely, and she could massage him after work feeling competent, loving, and secure in the knowledge that she was a good mother and her baby felt safe with her above all others. He settled into the massage and began to enjoy it, cooing and gazing at his mother, relaxing into the rhythmic strokes and the sound of her voice soothing him.

The Most Important Elements of Bonding and Attachment

The important elements that help form the bond between parent and infant include eye contact, skin contact, vocalization, the baby's responses to the parent, the activation of maternal and paternal hormones by contact with the baby, temperature regulation, and the immunizing bacteria and antibodies transferred to the baby by close contact with the parents.

While all of these elements come into play during the massage routine, the vital elements which strengthen bonds are eye contact, skin contact, vocalization, and communication—the baby's responses to the parent as well as the "dance" of learning intimately about one another.

Eye Contact

Eye contact is one of the most powerful communication systems we have. Between parent and infant, it is a vital connecting link. Parents seem compelled to get into a face-to-face position with their newborns and to gaze into their eyes. New parents croon to their babies, "Come on, now—open your eyes. Are you going to look at me?" Delighted exclamations follow when the infant makes eye contact. Parents report that they first feel very close to their babies when eye contact is made. The baby's visual system is biologically programmed to search out the contrasts in the bull's-eye shapes of the parent's eyes and nipples. Maternal hormones darken the areola during pregnancy, perhaps to help attract the baby's gaze. Experts speculate that eye contact may be a powerful cue to the infant's physiological system; the message received by the brain allows it to shut down the production of stress hormones initiated during childbirth. During a massage, the infant is positioned face to face with the parent, and the quality of interaction provides a lot of positive feedback, via eye contact, for parent and baby, continually reinforcing the message that it is "okay to relax now."

Skin Contact

Mothers seem to instinctively stroke their babies after birth, bringing myelination to the nerves and awakening the senses. Touch is a powerful element in human bonding. People in love, children forming friendships, even people who have acquired a new pet will spend extra time in close contact until the bond is secure. Animals raised without touch grow up to be antisocial and aggressive, and they tend to abuse and neglect their own young. Neurologist Richard Restak, author of *The Infant Mind*, comments on the importance of touch:

> *The infant turns toward the mother. How will she respond? Will she touch him? Will she turn away? How simple the situation, how seemingly devoid of content and importance. But we are deceived by the sim-*

plicity of this exchange which takes place within seconds but endures for decades. The mother turns toward her infant and touches him. Neither party speaks. Who could ever have guessed that simply touching another human being could be so important.

Vocalization

A third element in the dance of bonding is vocalization. From the moment he first responded to sound at around seven months gestation, your infant has been listening to your voice. His body moves in rhythm with your speech patterns, and the high-pitched tone you use when talking to him is particularly sweet to his ears. During his massage, you might sing a song or tell a story. He will come to associate certain sounds with the massage. Repeat his name and use the word *relax* to gently teach him how to release tension. (We'll cover this more in Chapter 5.)

Infant massage helps enhance the bond begun at birth. A baby learns to enjoy the wonderful comfort and security of loving and being loved. He acquires knowledge about his own body as his parent shows him how to relax a tense arm or leg, or helps him to release painful gas. His parent looks into his eyes, sings, talks soothingly, and gently strokes his skin. Thus, each day, the dance of bonding begins all over again.

"I feel much closer to my baby and more in tune with her body," says Debbie, mother of three-month-old Kelly. "Knowing that she is growing so fast, it is precious to be able to keep in touch with her little body and experience her growth day by day. I think she feels closer to me also, and there is a real trust developing because of our daily massage. I want to treasure her infancy with all its joys and problems. Massage is a wonderful way for me to do that. The benefits to my baby—physically and emotionally—are extra gifts."

Getting to Know Each Other

Regular massage provides a time for a parent to become intimately acquainted with the baby's body language, her rhythms of communication, her thresholds for stimulation, and how her body looks and feels when tense or at ease.

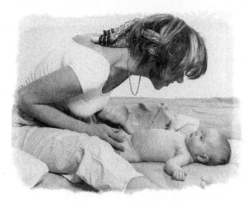

Bonding research also points out that parents feel closer to their infants if they can evoke a positive response from a specific series of actions. Massage, which combines intimacy, communication, play, and caregiving, can greatly enhance a parent's feeling of competence. Setting aside a time for touching and nurturing through massage, a parent sends her baby a very special message that says, "I love you and want to communicate with you, and you alone." From all my work, I can say that most babies do indeed get the message! My own children, grown adults now, continue to benefit from the daily massage routines we had when they were babies. They are affectionate, compassionate, well-rounded human beings. Our closeness has remained throughout their growing years, even the teens and early twenties, when they had to break away to create their own identities and their own paths in life. Though we have had our share of communication breakdowns, we always come back to each other with love—mending, reattaching, and becoming more close and understanding of one another. Our commitment to our family bonds is unbreakable, and I can say unequivocally that I attribute this closeness, our commitment to each other, to our early experiences in building strong attachments through loving, responsive massage.

DELAYED BONDING

Given the appropriate tools and encouragement, a parent and baby can certainly compensate if their bonding has been postponed by separation. If you were not able to establish intimate, affectionate bonds with your baby early on, don't despair. The beauty of the human species is that we have a marvelous ability to overcome setbacks and learn new patterns. If you are aware of the importance of these bonds, you can find ways to consciously assist nature.

An infant who avoids eye contact, who is stiff and doesn't mold to your body, may need some extra attention and help to begin to trust and form the attachments he needs for healthy development. Some of the ideas in Chapter 14 may help you. A daily massage can begin to recreate the elements of bonding that help you get in sync with one another. You may have to start with very little—perhaps only five minutes—and gradually increase as he begins to accept both your stroking and eye contact. Spending a little extra time carrying him, sleeping with him, taking baths with him, and playing with him when he is active and alert can also help. Whatever activities involve touching, talking, eye contact, and affection are the activities you can focus on. But go slowly. Some parents, in their anxiety at having missed the so-called early "bonding window," overcompensate by overstimulating and stressing their baby with too much, too fast. Allow the baby to lead, giving your attention, affection, eye contact, cuddling, carrying, and soothing in ways he can accept.

Some parents find this re-creation of bonding difficult because of an overload of stress or depression caused by separation from their infant. If you feel stressed or depressed, get help now. Counseling can

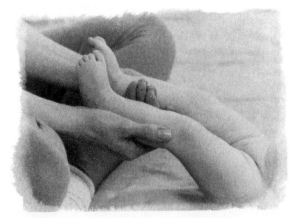

help a great deal; giving voice to pain is an essential means to healing. A counselor or psychotherapist can also help you find ways to deal with stress that you may not have thought about. For your baby's sake, for a long-term healthy relationship between the two of you, outside help can be invaluable.

In other chapters, we will discuss adoption, fostering, prematurity, and other special situations. Each of these will require a different approach to massage, but none rule it out as part of your parenting routines.

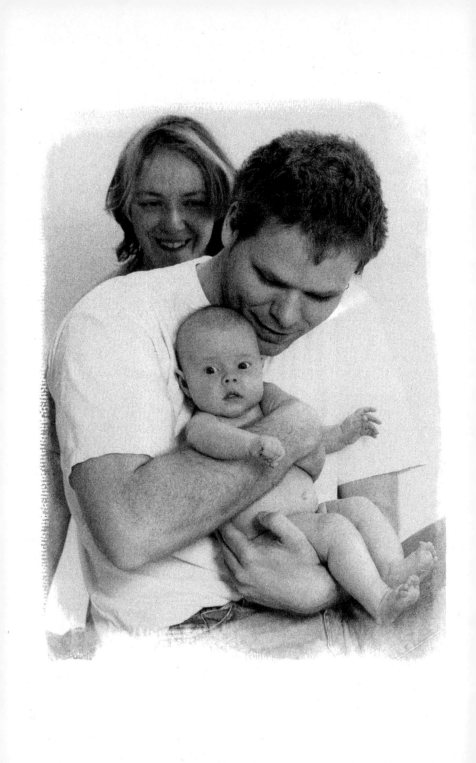

Chapter 4

Especially
for Fathers

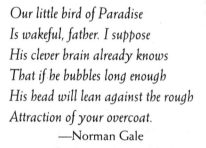

Our little bird of Paradise
Is wakeful, father. I suppose
His clever brain already knows
That if he bubbles long enough
His head will lean against the rough
Attraction of your overcoat.
 —Norman Gale

DAD, GET INVOLVED RIGHT FROM THE START

FATHERS TODAY take an increasingly active interest in the care and nurturing of their infants. The image of the clumsy, frightened father who hands the baby over to his wife until the child reaches a later, more playful age is fast becoming the exception rather than the rule.

In spite of this eagerness to participate in the baby's care right from the beginning, a new father may encounter logistical problems. His time may be limited to evenings and weekends. He may be tired after work. He may have to face the added stress of coping with basic household maintenance and increased financial pressure. In addition, his wife may work outside the home, so she has the same stresses to cope with and perhaps the added complication of breastfeeding while still maintaining her work-related image and expectations.

In the first weeks after birth, a mother may be tired at the end of the day, and the baby may be fussy. Far from fitting some people's notion of a stay-at-home mom luxuriating in the playful company of her baby and soap operas on television, the new mother has task after task to perform throughout the day, with no breaks and little contact with other adults. Many tasks are repetitive—cleaning, washing, diapering, feeding, comforting, grocery shopping—and there's not the validation of a paycheck or a pat on the back from a supervisor. So when dad gets home from his job, most moms aren't necessarily cheery. One father, whose wife had died, said he thought he had been very involved with his children before, but, "I didn't know how removed I was until I had to do all the thousands and thousands of things it takes to raise a child."

DON'T WAIT FOR AN INVITATION

Dads, don't wait for an invitation to get involved with the care of your baby. At the hospital, birthing center, or home, during the first few days, don't let well-meaning aunts or grandmothers push you out of the way. Ask the nurse or midwife or grandmother how to change, burp, take the temperature, and bathe your baby. If you and your partner have agreed, learn how to feed the baby. (Even breastfed babies can occasionally accept breast milk from a bottle.) If your partner complains about the way you do things, don't be defensive. Ask her to show you how she does it, and thank her. As one dad said, "After a while, she'll get tired of being the 'baby boss' and will relinquish more and more control to you." Studies have shown that a father's sensitive caregiving predicts secure attachment and that a warm, gratifying marital relationship supports fathers' involvement with their babies.

Both parents can be hard pressed to find time for themselves and

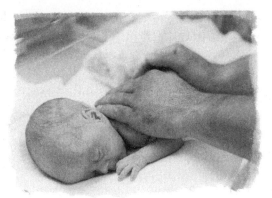

their relationship in addition to being good parents. A father may seem withdrawn at times when the mother and baby want and need just the opposite response. Moreover, the sometimes overwhelming responsibility of caring for the baby around the clock usually means, at least in the beginning, sleep deprivation for both parents.

These stressors give fathers a large barrier in learning to nurture their children with soft and gentle care. So does their lack of learned "maternal" behavior: because most men have not grown to manhood learning the same behaviors toward babies that most women do, they may need special help and encouragement in the beginning. But fathers can walk, rock, sing to, dance with, read to, and massage their babies as well as feed, change, and bathe them. Many people don't realize that fathers, too, have "parenting hormones" that are activated by close contact with their infants.

Psychologist Tom Daly comments, "In the process of giving the massage, fathers get to know their children in an extraordinary way. They connect with a deep part of the child and with a deep part of themselves—their nurturing side. Boys, by and large, are conditioned to suppress this part by the age of nine, but working with infants in this way opens up that old place. Dads find they are great nurturers when given a safe situation in which their manhood is not compromised."

When their fathers give children extra attention, he notes, the children have more self-confidence and exhibit more creativity. "Men and manhood are changing," he says. "Let us continue to get fathers more seriously involved in child rearing. Infant massage is a golden opportunity to assist in this transformation. The world is a better place every time an infant is massaged, and men need to be part of this."

NURTURANT MEN, SUCCESSFUL WOMEN: YOU CAN HELP

Children benefit immensely from affectionate interaction with both parents. "A warm, affectionate father-son relationship can strengthen a boy's masculine development," says Dr. Michael Lamb, author of *The Role of the Father in Child Development*. "A nurturant father is a more available model than a non-nurturant father. The nurturant father's behavior is more often associated with affection and praise and it acquires more reward value. Thus a boy with a nurturant father has more incentive to imitate his father than a boy with a non-nurturant father."

Girls, too, need wholesome bonds with their fathers. The Berkeley Longitudinal Study indicates that the women who were most healthy and well adjusted as adults grew up in homes with two loving, involved parents. The most successful women had fathers who valued femininity and encouraged competency, who were both warm and affectionate with their daughters and supportive of their efforts toward independence.

Massage is a quality experience for parents and infants, from which both benefit immensely. The baby learns that Daddy can touch him gently and lovingly, that Daddy, too, is someone he can count on to help meet his physical and emotional needs. A father who realizes these qualities in himself as a result of the massage experience is certain to have his confidence as a parent substantially boosted.

The most important process that evolves from regular massage between a father and his newborn is bonding. Just as breastfeeding provides consistent reinforcement of the bonding process for mothers—with its cuddling, skin contact, and face-to-face communication—so massaging can be just the thing to keep a father literally "in touch" with his baby. Fathers who massage their babies regularly throughout infancy later recall that massage time with fondness.

"I'll never forget how my son would wiggle and smile when he heard the oil swishing in my hands," says Ron, father of seven-month-old Jason. "It's going to be fun to tell him about it when he gets older and to remind him of it when he has his own kids. Heck, maybe someday I'll massage his baby, too!"

As a new father, you may have to use some creativity to structure your time to allow for the twenty to thirty minutes you will need to massage your baby. The best time is usually the morning of your day off, when you can relax unhurriedly. After learning the basic techniques from your wife, this book, or a class, you should be alone with your baby for the massage. It is better not to have both parents massaging the baby at once, as this can give your infant mixed signals and make him uncomfortable.

In the beginning, proceed very gently, massaging only the legs or back. You may have a sense of being too strong or too inexpert to massage your baby, your hands too big or rough. Nearly everyone is a little clumsy and nervous in the beginning. Start by gently placing your hands over your baby's back and feeling relaxation and love flow through your hands to your baby. You need not even move your hands in the beginning; just feel the connection between the two of you, and concentrate on relaxing your body and letting your love go to him. When that feels more comfortable, you can begin a simple stroking, stopping now and then to just hold and relax. Remember to make all your movements very smooth and slow, almost like slow motion. Talk or sing softly, make eye contact when baby is ready, and in general follow the baby's rhythms of communication. As time goes on and your baby becomes more familiar with your touch, you may want to spend more time and move on to other parts of the body, developing your own special massage techniques. For more ideas and helpful hints, please read on, for this book is meant for you as well.

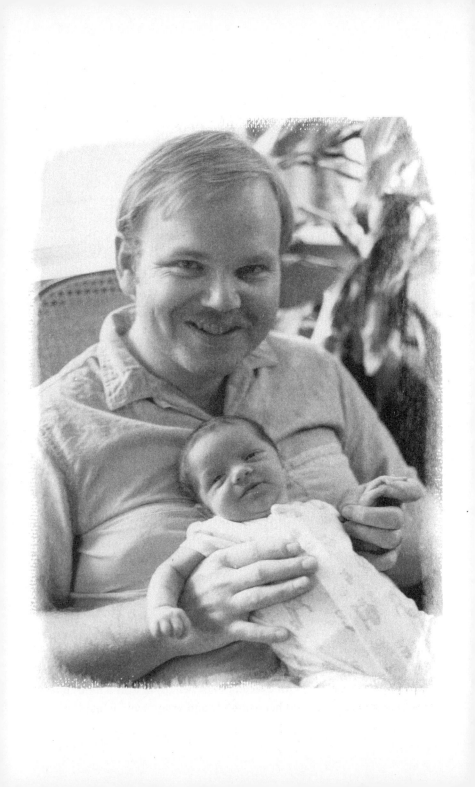

Chapter 5

Helping Baby
(and You)
Learn to Relax

There was a child went forth every day,
And the first object he look'd upon,
that object he became.
— Walt Whitman

VISUALIZE A RELAXED BABY, A RELAXED PARENT

CLOSE YOUR EYES for a moment, and picture your baby. What do you see? Is she awake or sleeping? Crying? Active or placid? Tense or relaxed? Chubby or thin? How does your mental image of her compare with the way she really is right now?

Often we unconsciously form images of ourselves and others, including our children, that are based upon limited experience. For instance, my second baby was ill and hospitalized just after she was born. She came home with a clean bill of health, but for a long time I subconsciously pictured her as fragile and weak. Even when I realized that I still carried my early fears and projected them to her, it was difficult to change that image. It had become a habitual way of thinking. These habits can directly affect those we think about, especially our children, who depend upon us for a clear reflection of themselves.

As parents' thinking is translated into words and actions, a baby adopts them as her own. Positive visualizations and affirmations can help free us from limiting concepts and give our infants feedback to develop to their full potential. The daily massage is a perfect opportunity to practice positive imagery and verbal feedback. As you massage your baby, picture her relaxing, opening, and letting go of tension. Visualize her happy and healthy. Try to picture her internal organs as you massage; see her heart beating, her lungs healthy, her intestinal system functioning smoothly. Imagine the blood as it moves through her veins and arteries. See your massage facilitating the blood flow to her arms and legs. Praise her relaxation, her beautiful smile, the softness of her skin. Here are a few examples of statements that help babies adopt positive attitudes about themselves:

> "How nice and soft your tummy is!"
> "I can feel the gas bubbles moving. Can you help push them out?"
> "You are learning to relax your legs. That's wonderful!"
> "Ah, so relaxed, so loose. You feel so happy now."
> "Sarah helps Mommy massage. Such a big girl!"

ARE YOU RELAXED?

The first few months of your baby's life are happy and exciting, but they can also be stressful. Right now, take an inventory of your body. Which areas are tense? Are you breathing deeply and fully? Perhaps you are holding your baby, nursing or walking about as you read. Is your baby fussy? When he cries, what happens to your body? Do you tense up, hold your breath, or breathe shallowly? If your baby is sleeping, are you anxious or restive, partially alert for his cries?

The miraculous changes you have undergone during pregnancy and delivery, the demands of caring for a new baby, and the lack of sleep and quiet time all add up to tension and anxiety, which can become habitual in the early weeks and months of parenthood. Your baby's daily massage offers a time to relax and unwind. In fact, a relaxed state of mind is essential.

At one time or another, every mother has felt tense and nervous, and in spite of her best efforts the baby begins to fuss and cry. Babies are wonderfully sensitive little beings who pick up every nuance of your communication. If you say "relax" with a furrowed brow, the baby will get both messages, but the furrowed brow is much more meaningful to him than your words.

Perhaps your baby has a fussy period during the day or evening. An hour or so before it usually begins, massage him to provide him with an outlet for built-up tensions. A simple fifteen-minute massage will be a welcome respite from the fussy baby—tense mother cycle.

In my son's early infancy, I discovered that massaging him, followed by taking a warm bath together, helped both of us avoid late afternoon irritability. In the summertime, a massage in the warm morning sun and a splash in the wading pool (made warm by adding hot water from the kitchen) gave me time for quiet, observant meditation and afforded my baby a wonderful sensory experience.

CONTROLLED BELLY BREATHING

In the last several years of my own practice and teaching, I have developed a technique I call Controlled Belly Breathing, which I do upon waking and again as I go to sleep at night. This practice can be very beneficial in relaxing and releasing tension, either to get ready for your day or to prepare for a restful night's sleep. It can be very helpful when your baby is ill and you are not able to get the sleep you need, or as a way to stay flowing with the everyday chaos that a family naturally brings with it.

I suggest you give this a try for at least a month, to see if it makes a difference in your life. Controlled Belly Breathing is easy to do and easy to incorporate into your routine, and if someday you wish to make a practice of daily meditation or prayer, this is wonderful preparation. And you can use it at any time, practicing in the car, on a bus, while cooking, before a meeting, virtually anywhere. It is especially helpful in preparation for potentially stressful events like dental work or surgery, and before something or someone comes at you with confrontive energy. (Many therapists recommend similar practices for people who have anxiety disorders or panic attacks.) You can use it when your child's behavior has you at the end of your rope, and you are so tired and upset you don't know what to do. You can also use it just before the massage routine, as a way of calming yourself and focusing on your love for your baby. Here's how it works:

1. Sit anywhere you like, with your back relatively straight. Your eyes can be open or closed. Breathe out, releasing all the air in your lungs.

2. Now slowly breathe in, through your nose, to a count of four (*1 and 2 and 3 and 4 and*).

3. Slowly release the air from your lungs at the same pace (*1 and 2 and 3 and 4 and*).

4. Repeat the entire in-out cycle for three minutes, timing yourself with a clock.

You will notice a slight pause at the end of each cycle, in and out. Let it be there. Don't force the technique, but imagine that the air is "breathing you." Breathe from the very bottom of your belly, allowing your belly to expand as the air comes in and contract as it goes out. During this time, you may say to yourself "relax" or any other word that comes to mind that helps you relax your body and release your mind of worries, cares, and lists. Notice any part of your body that is tense, and consciously relax that area. Some people like to say "slow down," others "let go," but you can simply use the counting as described above if you like.

TOUCH RELAXATION

One of the best things a parent can do for her child is to teach her to help herself. The ability to relax completely is a skill we all could use, and the earlier your child learns it, the more naturally it will come when she needs it. One of the benefits of daily massage for my children is the relaxed way they carry themselves today. They were ideal "demonstration models" in my classes because they knew how to relax, even as active toddlers. Children who have been taught Touch Relaxation techniques in infancy continue to respond as they get older.

The techniques of Touch Relaxation were extremely useful for my children's growing-up years. My eight-year-old daughter was having several teeth pulled in preparation for orthodontia. It was a frightening and painful experience. From the dentist's waiting room, I could hear her cries. I went to her and insisted that the dentist allow me to stay with her during the procedure. He was skeptical, but because she was so upset, he was willing to give it a try. I sat down beside her and began massaging her hands and using the gentle rolling, patting massage techniques I had developed for babies. I spoke to her in the high-pitched "mommy" voice I had used in her infancy, and I had her take a few deep breaths, close her eyes, and imagine she was floating on a cloud with the warm sun shining on her. She instantaneously relaxed her entire body, and the dentist was able to proceed without any further difficulty. I told her that each time she needed to relax more deeply, her kitten, Blackie, would come and rub against her leg. When I sensed her getting tense, I would quietly say, "Here comes Blackie," and massage her hand, and her body would go limp again. Physical stresses such as illness or injury, emotional stresses such as the first day of school or the loss of a pet, environmental tension such as the transition to a new home—all are situations in which relaxation techniques are invaluable.

How to Use Touch Relaxation

Touch Relaxation techniques—used between strokes, between sets of strokes, and after finishing the massage—are simple and easy to do. They fit in beautifully with the massage routine, but can also be done at other times. If you attended childbirth preparation classes, you may remember how you consciously rehearsed relaxing each part of your body. You will be using a similar principle with your baby, calling her attention to an area, showing her how to relax it, then giving her positive feedback as she learns.

For example, let's say you are beginning to massage the baby's leg, and it appears stiff and tense. Take the leg gently in your hands, encompassing and molding your hand to your baby's leg. Feel a heavy relaxation in your hand as it conforms to your baby's skin. Now, gently bounce the leg, repeating in a soft voice, "Relax," stressing and elongating the vowel sounds we spoke of in Chapter 2 ("*Reeee-laaaaax*"). Use the same tone each time you say this. As soon as you feel any relaxation in the muscles, give the baby some feed-

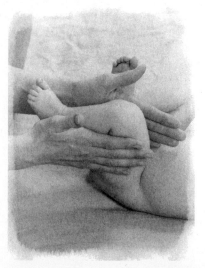

back, saying, "Wonderful! You relaxed your leg," and offer a smile and a kiss. The same thing can be done with other parts of the body. To loosen up the tense area, use very gentle rolling, bouncing, encompassing motions, giving positive feedback when you get a favorable response. Not only will this help the baby focus her attention on her own body so that later she knows how to relax herself, it will also help her to associate your touch with the positive benefits of relaxation. In Chapter 13, we will discuss how to use these benefits throughout your baby's childhood years.

RESTING HANDS

Sometimes at the beginning, especially with a medically fragile, premature, or colicky baby, and at different times during the massage, it is helpful to use a simple holding technique. My favorite, developed by infant massage instructor trainer Helena Moses, is called Resting Hands. Warming your hands, you simply place them on the baby, wherever you are. It may be holding the baby's legs, resting your hands on her belly or chest, holding her arms, or rest-

ing your hands on her back. Let your hands go very heavy and warm. Intentionally relax your own body, and slow down your breathing. Imagine healing and relaxation flowing through your 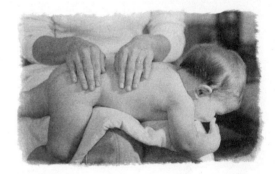 hands to your baby. See if you can warm up your hands, just using the power of your mind and deeply relaxing your body.

I believe every massage should begin this way, to help both parent and baby slow down and relax into the gentle love of conscious, healthy touch.

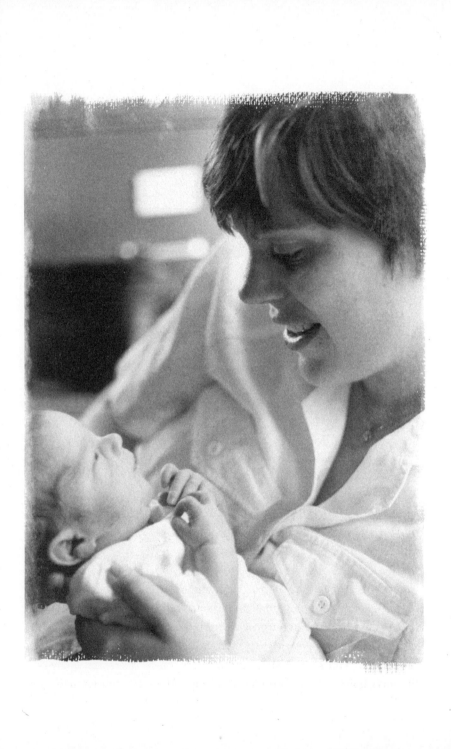

Chapter 6

Music and
Massage

Upon what Instrument are we two spanned?
And what player has us in his hand?
O sweet song. .
—Rainer Maria Rilke

YOUR VOICE can be an important part of your baby's massage. By talking softly, humming, or singing, you create an atmosphere of calm. This verbal communication will also help you keep your mind in the present and your attention on your baby.

Singing is a wonderful way to relax. Sing to your baby anytime—while changing diapers, feeding, rocking, or walking. You will discover there are some songs your baby loves to hear again and again. His sense of musical discrimination will astound you!

Familiar lullabies from your own childhood would fit in beautifully here. Think of your grandmother's music box that played Brahms's lullaby or the wonderful, lilting "Alouette" you learned in

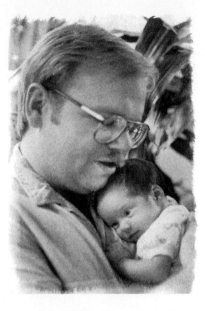

elementary school. Recall how your own mother sang "Go to Sleep, My Baby" to your younger brother or sisters, and do likewise with your baby.

In one study, parents were asked to sing a song of their choice in two ways. First, they would sing it in the way they would sing it to their baby, even though the baby was not present. Then, the parent would sing the same song to the baby herself. When other adults were asked to listen to these recordings, they could nearly always identify the song that was sung directly to the infant; these versions tended to be sung at a higher pitch, with much more emotional engagement, elongation of vowel sounds, and more slowly. Interestingly, the fathers sang more slowly to their infants than did the mothers.

This study helps confirm my earlier discussion of how babies respond to their parents' vocalization, when parents unconsciously make it easier for their babies to understand by elongating vowel sounds. So babies actually affect the way parents vocalize; there is a synchrony of interaction that is part of the dance of bonding. Singing is a wonderful way to soothe your baby and capture his attention.

Here are some folk lullabies from around the world. (Notice how most lullabies have many elongated vowel sounds in them.) Undoubtedly you have some family favorites to add to this collection. In "References and Recommendations," I have included a list of books and music that will help you utilize this wonderful tool in your practice of infant massage.

LULLABIES FROM AROUND THE WORLD

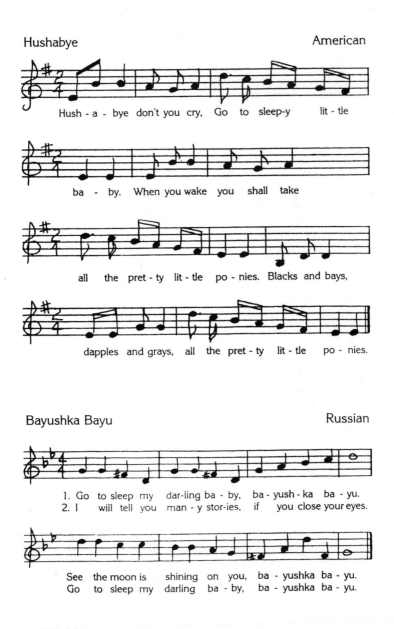

Hushabye   American

Hush - a - bye don't you cry, Go to sleep-y lit - tle

ba - by. When you wake you shall take

all the pret - ty lit - tle po - nies. Blacks and bays,

dapples and grays, all the pret - ty lit - tle po - nies.

Bayushka Bayu   Russian

1. Go to sleep my dar-ling ba - by, ba - yush - ka ba - yu.
2. I will tell you man - y stor-ies, if you close your eyes.

See the moon is shining on you, ba - yushka ba - yu.
Go to sleep my darling ba - by, ba - yushka ba - yu.

Schlaf, Kindlein, Schlaf

German

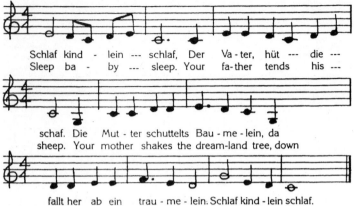

Schlaf kind - lein --- schlaf, Der Va - ter, hüt --- die ---
Sleep ba - by --- sleep. Your fa-ther tends his ---

schaf. Die Mut - ter schuttelts Bau - me - lein, da
sheep. Your mother shakes the dream-land tree, down

fallt her ab ein trau - me - lein. Schlaf kind - lein schlaf.
falls a lit - tle dream for thee. Sleep, ba - by sleep.

Dors, Mon Petit Enfant

French

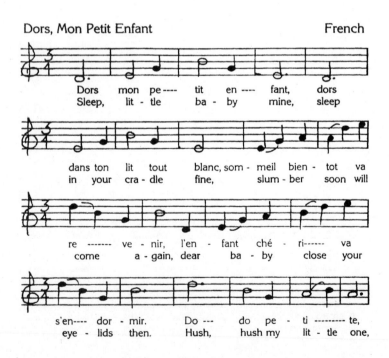

Dors mon pe---- tit en ---- fant, dors
Sleep, lit - tle ba - by mine, sleep

dans ton lit tout blanc, som - meil bien - tot va
in your cra - dle fine, slum - ber soon will

re ------- ve - nir, l'en - fant ché - ri------ va
come a - gain, dear ba - by close your

s'en---- dor - mir. Do --- do pe - ti -------- te,
eye - lids then. Hush, hush my lit - tle one,

54

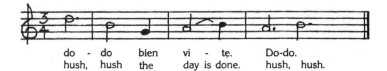

do - do bien vi - te. Do-do.
hush, hush the day is done. hush, hush.

Lullaby

Japanese

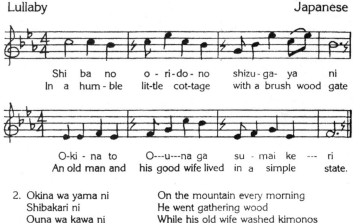

Shi ba no o - ri-do-no shizu - ga - ya ni
In a hum - ble lit-tle cot-tage with a brush wood gate

O-ki - na to O---u---na ga su - mai ke --- ri
An old man and his good wife lived in a simple state.

2. Okina wa yama ni   On the mountain every morning
   Shibakari ni   He went gathering wood
   Ouna wa kawa ni   While his old wife washed kimonos
   Kinu susugi.   In the river's flood.

Arrullo Mi Niño

Spanish

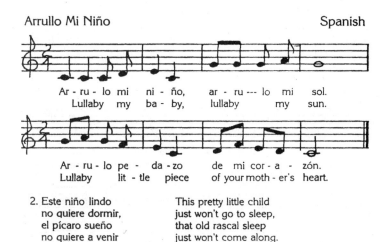

Ar - ru - lo mi ni - ño, ar - ru --- lo mi sol.
Lullaby my ba - by, lullaby my sun.

Ar - ru - lo pe - da - zo de mi cor - a - zón.
Lullaby lit - tle piece of your moth - er's heart.

2. Este niño lindo   This pretty little child
   no quiere dormir,   just won't go to sleep,
   el pícaro sueño   that old rascal sleep
   no quiere a venir   just won't come along.

55

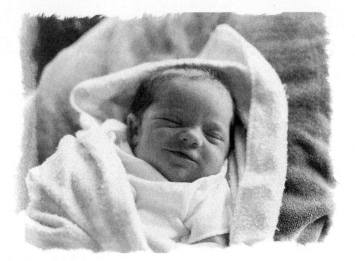

The following Bengali chant from India means "I love you, my dear baby." Its wonderfully soothing effect on babies has made it a favorite in our infant massage classes, and it has become nearly an "anthem" for the International Association of Infant Massage. The words are pronounced: *aaah-mee toe-mah-kay, bah-lo bah-shee baaaabeee.*

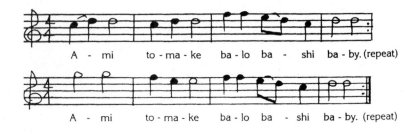

A - mi   to - ma - ke   ba - lo ba - shi   ba - by. (repeat)

A - mi   to - ma - ke   ba - lo ba - shi   ba - by. (repeat)

PLAY SOME MUSIC, TELL A STORY

If you are not comfortable singing, simply tell a story or talk about the massage as you go. It is the tone of your voice that is most important, not the quality of the words and music you project.

Fathers often find massage time to be a pleasant opportunity to play music they like for background music. Guitar music, pleasant rhythmic tunes that inspire smooth, slow movements, seem to work best. Perhaps you have some music in your household that would offer an accompaniment to your baby's massage. A soft symphony, a slow reggae melody, a raga of Indian sitar, angelic choir music, or the sound of ocean waves would all provide a beautiful background for your loving touch.

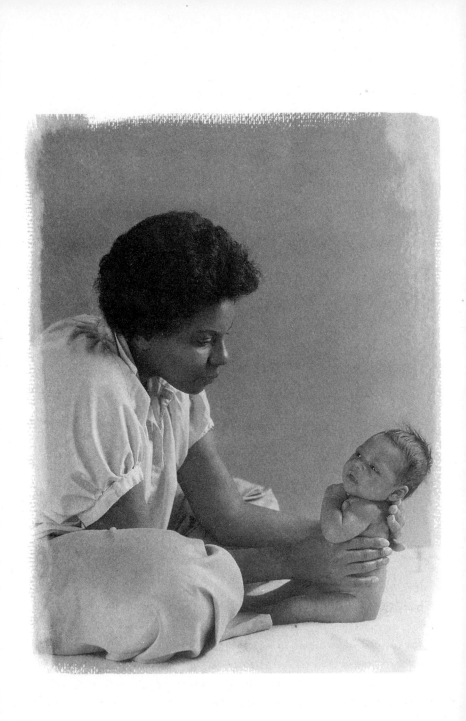

Chapter 7

Getting Ready

※

O young thing, your mother's lovely armful!
How sweet the fragrance of your body!
—Euripides

WHEN TO START

EVEN WITHOUT conscious awareness, a mother will usually begin massaging her baby, ever so gently, from the moment of birth. It is part of the bonding process—a biological urge to know her baby through all her senses.

The massage in this book can be started as soon as you desire. For the first six or seven months, your baby will benefit most from a daily massage. As your child becomes more active through crawling or walking, you may reduce it to once a week, as desired. Your toddler may enjoy a rubdown before bed or after bath time. In this case, you should certainly continue it. In Chapter 13, we will discuss what modifications you will need to make for your child's larger body and different needs.

WHAT TIME AND WHERE

Experiment to find the time and place that are best for you and your baby. Generally, the morning is a good time, when both of you have been fed and are ready for the day. But there are also advantages to afternoon and evening massages. For some babies, a massage before a nap is good for releasing that last bit of energy so they can sleep more soundly. For others, however, any stimulation is too much, and all they need is rest. For such a baby, give the massage after the nap. The evening is also a good time for some; if the baby is tired but not too cranky, it might help him to sleep. Your schedule must also be considered. You may work outside the home or have other small children to care for. The evening may be the best time for you, when the day's work is done and your partner can watch the other children. A massage will give you and your new baby the time together you both deserve.

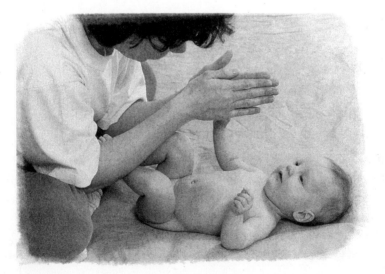

In the early months, a delightful routine is to massage the baby, then fill a warm bath and take her in with you. The bath becomes a wonderfully relaxing experience, and your baby may even fall asleep in your arms. To her, the experience is rather like a "womb with a view," in that she floats in the womblike warm water, yet at the same time she can see you as you support her with comfort and security. She may cry when you take her out of the tub (it can remind her of the shock of going from womb to the cold outer world), but usually some cuddling and/or nursing will quiet her.

You're probably wondering how both of you can get out of the tub safely and without becoming chilled. First, be sure the bathroom is nice and warm. Keep an infant seat covered with towels next to the tub, and when you are ready to get out, put her in the seat, swaddling her with the towels. Then you can get out and dry off, and perhaps you can both crawl into bed for a nap, or get going with your day.

From about six months of age, when bath time becomes more of a playtime for your baby, the massage works better afterward, when she is a little more tired and is almost ready for a nap. The massage can help her release that last bit of tension so she can sleep deeply.

Always massage in a warm, quiet place. In the summer, try experiencing the warm morning sun, the sounds of birds, and the smell and feel of the summer air. Take the baby to the beach and massage her with the sound of the water nearby. But take your time. Your baby is only a baby once.

WARMTH

Peter Wolff, a well-known pediatrician and researcher who completed countless studies of newborns and their behavior, observed that temperature has an important effect on the amount of time babies sleep and on their crying. Babies kept at warmer temperatures, he found, cried less and slept more than those subjected to cooler environments.

Rudolf Steiner, philosopher, scientist, educator, and propounder

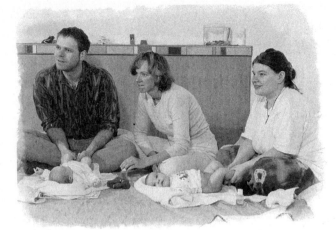

of Waldorf Education, also stressed the importance of keeping babies warm. He asserted that the formative forces, both physical and spiritual, that work to help babies' bodies and souls grow properly need this warmth to be effective.

I have observed that babies in our infant massage classes, especially those under three months of age, are much more comfortable, startle less, and relax more easily if they are kept quite warm. If your room is cool, you may want to place a small, safe, portable heater in the room. Or you can wrap a baby-size warm-water bottle in a towel and tuck it under the blanket near the baby's feet for the massage. The room should be warm enough so that you can wear light clothing and still feel warm. Remember, your baby has much less bulk to warm him, and without clothing he could be chilled, which can cause fussing.

POSITIONING

Find a comfortable sitting position for massaging your baby. Your back should be relatively straight, with most of your movement coming from your lower back as a center. You can sit on the floor or on a bed cross-legged with your baby in front of you on a pillow or blanket; some baby-care companies even make pillows especially for this purpose. Remember to bring the baby as close to you as possible, with his bottom firmly resting against your crossed legs.

CRADLE POSE

During the newborn period, the position used in India, which I call the Cradle Pose, can work wonderfully if your body can do it without discomfort. Here's how: Sit on the floor with legs stretched out, back supported against a wall or furniture. Now bend your knees slightly outward, touching the soles of your feet together slightly. Pad the area between your knees with thick blankets, making an indentation in the middle for your baby. Place the baby in the "cradle" of your legs, facing you. This position helps the baby feel more securely positioned and helps conserve warmth. Because babies have the tonic neck reflex for the first four to six months, it is natural, when lying flat, for them to look off to the side. The angle of your legs in Cradle Pose helps tip the baby up slightly toward you. Placing the baby's head at the arches of your feet will help keep his head aligned for eye contact.

You can give a massage in other positions as well. You can use a changing table, all the better if the table can be lowered so you can sit in a chair and relax. Massage can be given in sections and at various times. After changing the diaper, you can massage your baby's legs, arms, or back, and use Touch Relaxation and Resting Hands to reinforce your regular massage sessions.

WHAT YOU NEED

Assemble massage oil (which we will talk about next), towels, a few extra diapers, and a change of clothes for baby. You should wear something comfortable that you wouldn't mind getting a little soiled. Before beginning, remember to warm the area, wash your hands, remove your jewelry, and relax your body.

WHICH OILS, AND WHY?

As your hands glide over your baby's delicate skin, the last thing you want to do is to create any sort of friction. Using an oil eliminates friction.

Most of the time, you will need a light natural oil. The only exception might be where the baby's skin is very dry, and an oil-based massage lotion that absorbs into the skin may help soften more easily. But for regular massages, oil is better than lotion because lotion tends to soak into the skin quite rapidly, which means you constantly have to stop the massage in order to reapply it.

The primary benefit of oil is that it makes the movement smoother on your baby's skin. As you are working, you apply the oil to your hands. I tell parents in my classes to pour a little less than a teaspoon of oil into one palm, then rub the palms together to warm the oil; do not pour the oil directly onto your baby's body. As you massage, reapply as necessary. There should be just enough oil to make your movements smooth without being overly slick.

For a number of reasons, I prefer cold-pressed fruit and/or vegetable oils to mass-produced, commercially advertised "baby oils." What we put on our skin is absorbed into the body and circulates throughout, carried by lymph, a liquid like blood that cleanses the body of toxins and carries away waste. If we are going to use a topical application on our little ones, we quite naturally want to use a product that will nourish them rather than one that may actually rob them of vital nutrients, being nonorganic and petroleum based. Most "baby oils" are primarily made of mineral oil. To make mineral oil, gasoline and kerosene are removed from crude petroleum by heating, in a method called functional distillation. By using sulfuric acid, applying absorbents, and washing with solvents and alkalis, hydrocarbons and other chemicals are then removed.

Not only is there no food value in this type of oil, but some nutritional authorities believe that mineral oil, when ingested, produces deficiencies of various vitamins, and they recommend against its use as a regular massage oil. When you are in the middle of the massage and your baby puts his hand in or near his mouth, you don't want to worry that a nonfood substance is passing into his delicate digestive system. Infants, whose brains and nervous systems are not fully developed, are particularly vulnerable to substances absorbed by the skin. Commercially produced mineral oils also dry the skin and clog its pores. Most modern pediatricians discourage their use for this reason alone. These oils were not made for regular massage, which encourages the absorption of whatever substance you are using. That substance, in my view, should be a food product that nourishes the skin.

In India mothers vary the oils they use by the season. In winter they use hardy mustard oil to conserve warmth. During the summer, they switch to coconut oil for cooling. Apricot kernel and almond oils are two of my personal favorites because of their light, smooth feel and the fact that they are absorbed readily. Such oils keep intact not only their vitamins and minerals but also their fatty acids, which contribute to healthy skin. Since these oils are nondrying, they nurture and moisturize the skin rather than deplete it. Try a "patch" test on your baby with any massage oil you select. If a rash develops, your baby could be sensitive to it, so you should switch to something else, such as canola, safflower, or avocado oil. Regular bathing keeps the baby's pores from clogging and rashes from developing.

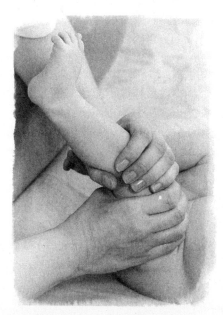

If the oil you select is enhanced with vitamin E, so much the better, since this vitamin has been shown to be especially good for the skin and has the added benefit of preserving the oil's freshness. If you use a plain vegetable oil, you may want to add a drop or two of vitamin E oil as a natural preservative. It is a natural antioxidant, which means it inhibits the product from rancidity. Cold-pressed oils keep the vitamin E intact, while heating and other refining procedures tend to destroy it.

Odor is an often overlooked part of the bonding process. An infant's olfactory system is ready to function as early as seventeen weeks gestation, so it must be an important function for the newborn. A highly refined sense of smell immediately following birth helps a baby distinguish his mother's chemical "signature." Unfortunately, we often assault our infant's senses with noxious smells and thus inhibit this means of bonding. For this reason, I recommend that you use an unscented oil for your newborn's massage. (In the Resources section, I list recommended sources for baby massage oils.)

THE MASSAGE TECHNIQUE: HOW MUCH PRESSURE?

Infant massage is not manipulative in the way adult massage by a professional massage therapist may be; there is no vigorous kneading. It is a gentle, firm, warm communication. A baby's muscles, which comprise only a quarter of her total body weight (as compared to almost half in adulthood), aren't developed enough to have knots of tension. Her body is so tiny that a gentle but firm effleurage is enough to stimulate circulation and tone the internal functions.

In the beginning, while you are learning and your baby is tiny, be soft and gentle. As your baby grows, your massage will grow firmer. Do not be afraid to touch her firmly. You will find she enjoys being handled and massaged in a manner that communicates your strength, love, and confidence. All of your strokes should be long, slow, and rhythmic, with just enough pressure to be comfortable but stimulating. Avoid stroking your baby with a fluttery, poking, or tickly touch. The massage given here should be done as much as possible with your whole hand molding to the baby's body with a gentle but firm pressure, just enough to encourage circulation and let your baby know he is in the hands of a strong, capable caregiver.

Dr. Tiffany Field, of the Touch Research Institute, notes: "Although infants, particularly premature infants, for example, may seem to be fragile, some pressure is needed for the massage to be effective. In our review of the infant massage literature we found that those who used light stroking did not report weight gain, for example, while those who used stroking with pressure reported weight gain."

I have found in my work with parents and babies that rather than having to caution parents to be gentle, I often need to encourage them to stroke the baby with a firm but gentle, rhythmic motion. Too tentative, soft, or ticklish massage is generally irritating to babies. They like to feel the strong, warm comfort of their parents' loving hands.

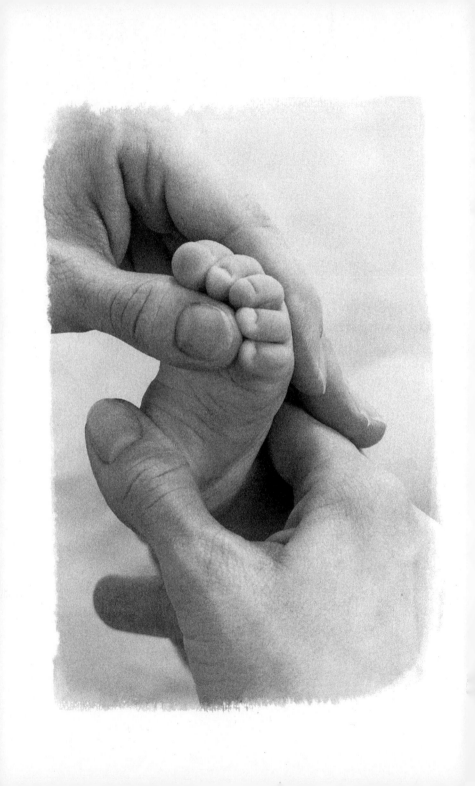

Chapter 8

How to Massage Your Baby

When from the wearying war of life
I seek release
I look into my baby's face
And there find peace.
　　　　　—Martha F. Crow

W HEN YOU have assembled your tools and have found a comfortable spot for the two of you, take a few minutes to sit quietly. Starting at the top of your head, relax every muscle in your
body as much as you can. Feel the wave of relaxation wash over
you, from your head to the tips of your toes.

Now gently let your head fall forward so that your chin
touches your chest. Slowly rotate your head, first clockwise, then
counterclockwise, stretching your neck so that your head sweeps in
complete, wide, slow circles. Feel all the muscles in your neck and
shoulders stretch and relax.

Now shrug your shoulders, up toward your ears. Hold them

there a few seconds, then release them downward. Repeat a few times. Rotate your shoulders forward, then backward, and shake them out, feeling your entire upper body and arms relax and center.

RELAX AND BREATHE FULLY

A harmonious mind parallels slow, deep, and regular breathing. As you massage your baby, breathe deeply and slowly so that your lungs fill with air down into your belly and then exhale completely. Once in a while, take an audible sigh, breathing in through your nose and exhaling through your mouth, at the same time you consciously relax your body. Your baby will feel this and eventually begin to imitate your relaxing sighs.

Before you undress your baby and begin the massage, get your body into the right position. This may be sitting on the floor cross-legged, with your baby in front of you, as close to you as possible. It may be sitting in a chair, or standing before a changing table, or sitting on a bed with your baby in front of you, again, as close as possible. Relax as much as you can from head to toe. Now breathe deeply, expanding your belly to take in as much air as possible. As you breathe out, blowing softly from your mouth, affirm, "I now let go of tension. My body is relaxed." Feel all traces of tension or anxiety leave your body. You are confident and centered.

With the next breath, as you gently blow air out after the in-breath, affirm, "I release all other thoughts and focus on my baby." Let all worries and plans leave your mind, like birds flying through a clear blue sky. You are here now—just you and your baby. You deserve this time together.

Breathe in deeply again, and while blowing out softly, affirm to yourself, "I am the gentle power of love, flowing through my hands to my baby." Visualize all the love you feel for your baby as a brilliant sun in the center of your heart. With each heartbeat, its warm radiance courses through your arms, into your hands, and over your baby as you begin the massage.

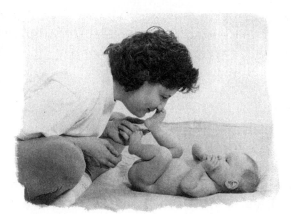

Greet your baby with your words, your smile, and your touch. Let her know her massage is about to begin.

REQUEST PERMISSION TO BEGIN

When you are relaxed, focused, and ready to begin, remove your baby's clothing and any jewelry you may have on—particularly rings and bracelets, or necklaces that may dangle and distract. If this is your first session, you may just want to remove the bottom half of his clothing, as I encourage you to begin with only the legs today. Do remove the diaper, though, and lightly cover the front with a loose cloth or diaper to protect yourself from mishaps.

In subsequent sessions, you can begin to add more strokes. It may take a few or many sessions before your baby enjoys a full body massage. You will know as you go along how much massage the baby wants and needs as you get to know the routine and your baby becomes comfortable with it.

As you remove his clothing, tell him that it is massage time, and give him a special "cue" that you are about to start. Here's how: Pour a small amount of massage oil into your palm. Now rub your palms together to warm them, saying, "It's time for massage." Your baby will hear the oil swishing between your hands and alert to the sound of the word *massage*. Show your palms to your baby, saying,

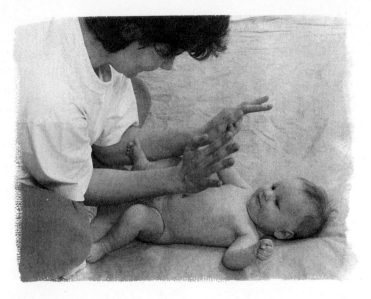

"May I massage you now?" The first time, of course, your baby doesn't know what is about to happen. But in subsequent sessions, this routine will become a cue to which he will respond.

How can you tell if your baby is saying, "No?" Usually the baby will throw hands up in a guarding motion, turn her head away, kick, and fuss. The baby may begin to hiccup, to flail her arms, and move her eyes around frantically.

If you get a "no," you may want to try warming up the space or covering him with a blanket; bring him closer to you, and lay your warm hands on his legs, using deep relaxation—the Resting Hands we talked about in Chapter 5. Then ask again. Often a small change in comfort is all that is necessary. Or maybe you need to relax more deeply. Think of things you could do to change the atmosphere to make it more warm and comfortable for your baby. If you still get a very clear "no!" wait for another time to try again. If the baby seems a little fussy but not definite, continue with the massage. Often a fussy baby will calm down and start enjoying the massage after you have finished a leg or two. The next time you massage, the experience will be more familiar, and the fussing may diminish.

This preparatory routine serves several important purposes. It lets the baby know that a new experience is about to begin, and it helps him to get ready for it. It also communicates—through your voice and your body language—respect for him. It says, "You are worthy of respect. You are in charge of your body, and people should ask your permission to interact with you in this way." Later, in Chapter 13, we will discuss how these early experiences can help your child know the difference between healthy and unhealthy touching as he grows older. Using these cues before beginning a massage now will help build the trust, respect, and values that will ensure a healthy life.

JUST THE TWO OF YOU

As you massage your baby, every movement of your body will be an expression of your love. Your strong, gentle touch, the rhythm you create, the way you move back and forth with each stroke, your eyes, your smile, and your voice are all as much a part of the experience as the massage itself. Gaze into your baby's eyes, and open yourself to the love you share. Relax, and begin your massage with a gentle contact of your baby's skin. Feel your hands, heavy,

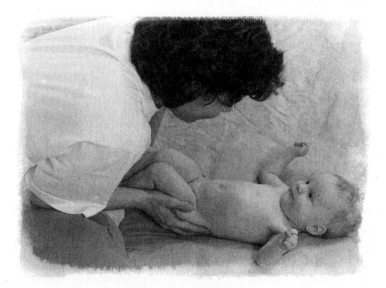

warm, and relaxed, supporting your baby. Unless otherwise indicated, repeat each stroke at least three to four times.

"May I Massage Your Legs and Feet?"

We begin with the legs and feet for several reasons. Babies reach out to the world with their legs and feet. Observe your baby closely when interacting with new people. Before making eye contact, most infants will wiggle their feet and legs. Indeed, you may detect a kind of sign language your baby uses with her feet to make contact with other people and establish trust. Even two babies brought into proximity will kick and wiggle their legs, as if conversing with each other with their feet!

The feet and legs are the least vulnerable part of your baby's body. If, right at first, you begin massaging her upper body, she may become tense and anxious. She will instinctively "close" her arms and legs to protect her vital organs. Beginning with the legs and feet gives her a chance to establish trust and accept the massage gradually.

For many babies, the legs and feet are the most pleasurable part of the massage. Thus, beginning with the legs will help baby to relax all over.

If your baby has been hospitalized for any reason, she probably received several heel sticks when hospital personnel drew blood for testing. Sensitivity in this area can remain long after the bruises have disappeared. If your baby seems to react with fear or displeasure when you begin to massage her foot, stop using the strokes and simply hold her foot gently in your palms, molding your hands to it. Use this holding technique for a few days to help her accept touch, then try stroking again.

The Indian and Swedish Milking strokes aid circulation to the feet and back toward the heart. The Squeeze and Twist and Rolling strokes help tone and relax the legs.

Massage one leg completely, then the other. Start by greeting your baby's legs with Resting Hands.

1. INDIAN MILKING.
Milk the leg with the inside edge of each hand (the part where your thumb and index finger are), encompassing the leg and molding the hands to it, one following the other. The opposite hand gently holds the ankle. The outside hand should move over the buttock; the inside hand moves inside the thigh and up the leg to the ankle.

Move in rhythmic strokes, with your lower back/pelvis as your center of gravity. Remember to use the bottom hand to keep your baby's pelvis on the floor, so that you do not lift the baby's body with your strokes.

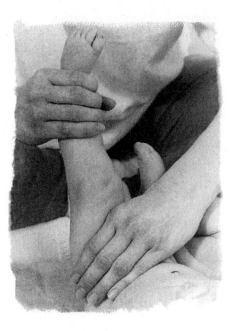

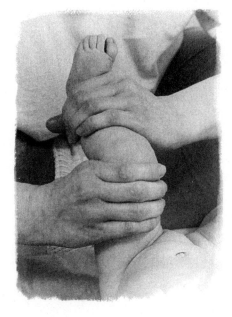

2. HUG AND GLIDE. Hold the leg with the inside edge of your hands (the part where your thumb and index finger are) facing upward. Keep your hands together so as not to twist the knee joint, and encompass the leg as much as possible. Stroke from the thigh to the ankle, gently turning in opposite directions, forward and back, squeezing very slightly. This stroke moves across the muscle and thus helps it relax.

3. THUMB OVER THUMB. Stroke your thumbs, one after the other, from the heel to the toes.

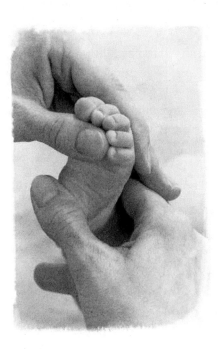

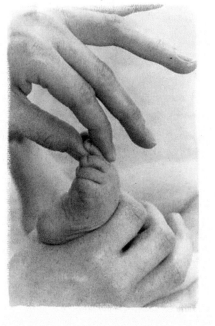

4. TOE ROLL. Squeeze and roll each toe.

There are seventy-two thousand nerve endings in each foot. The many theories of how foot massage works all agree that points on the feet connect with other body areas. Environmental stresses can cause imbalances in our system which we experience as colds, flu, ear infections, and so forth. Reflexologists (those who study and work with these points on the feet) say that by-products of these imbalances, uric acid and excess calcium, can calcify around nerve endings in the feet, blocking the flow of energy through the body. Foot massage, they say, moves this excess calcium and uric acid out, so that they are absorbed by the blood and lymph and eventually excreted out of the body.

5. UNDER TOES. With your forefinger, gently press the ball of the foot, just under the toes.

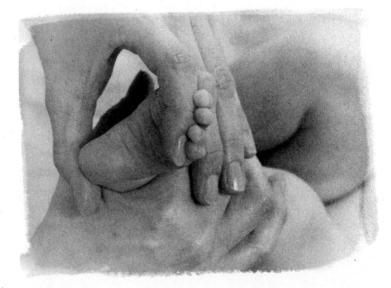

6. HEEL OF FOOT. With your forefinger, press the ball of the foot where the heel begins, and massage this area gently.

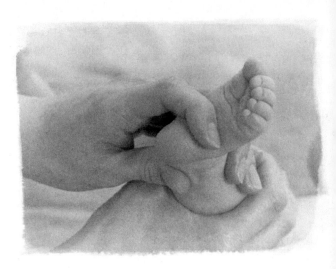

7. THUMB PRESS. Press in with your thumbs all over the bottom of the foot.

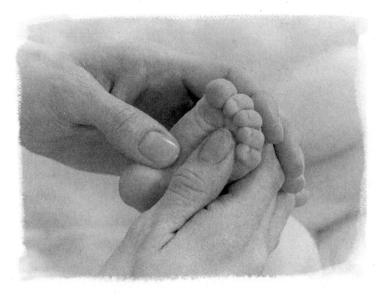

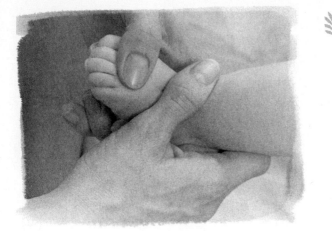

8. TOP OF FOOT. Using your thumbs, one after the other, stroke the top of the foot toward the ankle.

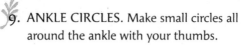

9. ANKLE CIRCLES. Make small circles all around the ankle with your thumbs.

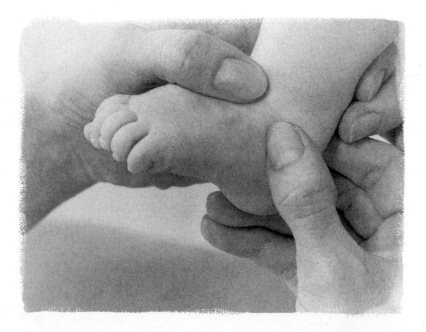

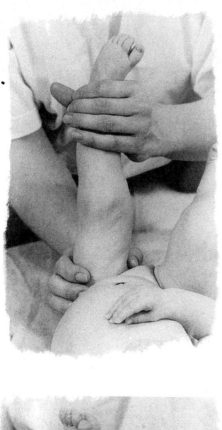

10. SWEDISH MILKING.
Milk the leg from ankle
to hip, stabilizing the
leg at the ankle, mov-
ing one hand on the
outside of the leg, then
the other on the inside.
Remember not to pull
the baby's body up off
the surface.

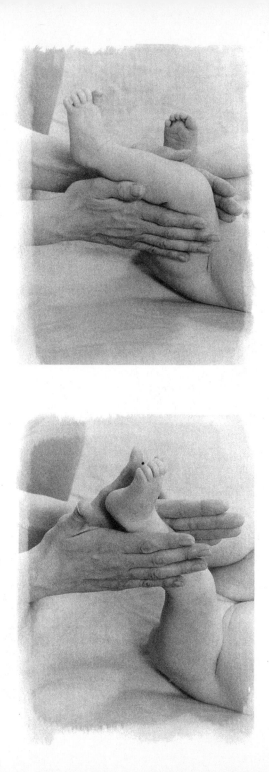

11. ROLLING.
Roll the leg between your hands from thigh to ankle. Most babies love this!

12. BOTTOM RELAXER.

After massaging each leg and foot, massage the buttocks with both hands in small circles, then stroke the legs to the feet, gently bouncing.

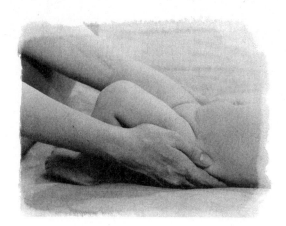

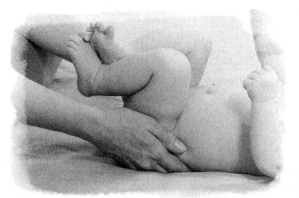

13. INTEGRATION.

Move both hands with a sweeping stroke from buttocks to feet. This integrates the legs with the torso and lets baby know you are moving to another part of the body.

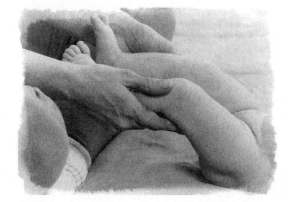

"May I Massage Your Tummy?"

The strokes for the stomach will tone your baby's intestinal system and help relieve gas and constipation. Most of the strokes end at the baby's lower left belly (your right). This is where the eliminative part of the intestine is located. The purpose is to move gas and intestinal matter toward the bowel. Always stroke from the rib cage down, and use a clockwise motion for circular strokes. If you have a colicky baby, a special routine is given in Chapter 10.

1. RESTING HANDS. Start by making contact with your baby's tummy, laying your hand on the belly with a heavy, warm, relaxed feeling, letting your baby know it is time to massage the belly.

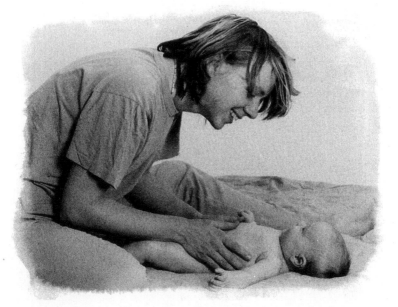

2. WATER WHEEL PART A. Make paddling strokes on your baby's tummy, one hand following the other, as if you were scooping a depression into sand. Keep your hands molded to the baby's tummy. Do not use the edge of your hand. Repeat about six times.

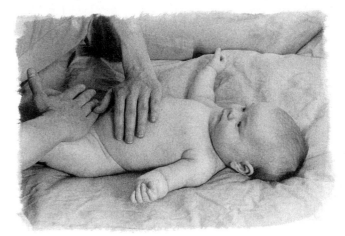

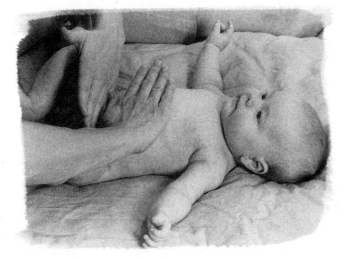

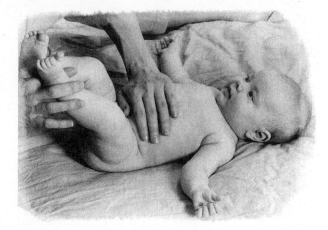

3. WATER WHEEL PART B. Hold your baby's legs up with one hand, grasping the ankles gently. Your baby's body should be close to you, hips anchored firmly on the floor. Do not lift the baby's body. With your other hand, repeat the paddling motion. This will relax the stomach and permit you to extend the massage a little more deeply.

Another way to hold your baby's legs up for this stroke is to cross your right hand under the baby's left leg and hold on to the right, so your right arm holds up both legs. Stroke with the left hand. (You can reverse this if your dominant hand is the right.)

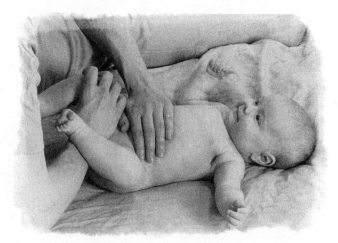

4. THUMBS TO SIDES. With thumbs flat at the baby's navel, push out to the sides. Be sure you use the flat thumb, and do not poke.

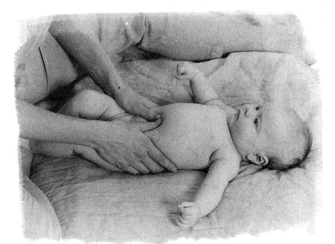

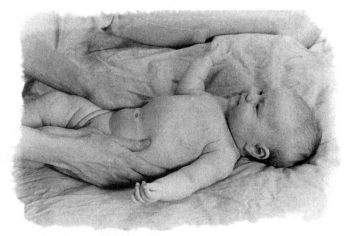

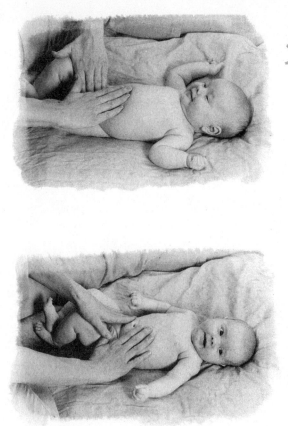

5. SUN MOON.
Your left hand
strokes in a full
circle, moving
clockwise start-
ing at your left
(7 o'clock). As
the left hand is
making the
lower part of the
circle, the right
hand makes a
half moon
above, just
below the rib
cage, stroking
from baby's right
to left (your left
to right), like an
upside-down **U**.

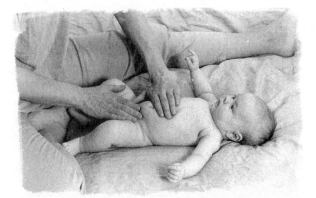

6. I LOVE YOU.
As you go through this series of strokes, say "I love you!" in a high-pitched, cooing tone. Your baby will love it! First, make

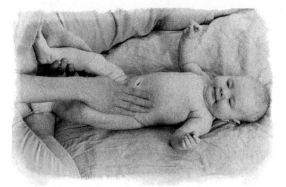

a single I-shaped stroke with your right hand on baby's left belly several times, pressing the pads of your fingers straight down from baby's rib cage (*Iiiiiiiiiiii*).

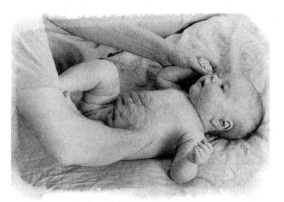

Next, make a backward, sideways L going from your left to right and then down (*looooooove*).

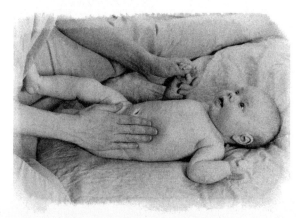

Make an upside-down U, going from your left to right (from baby's right to left), with the upper part of the stroke under the rib cage (*yooooooooooou!*).

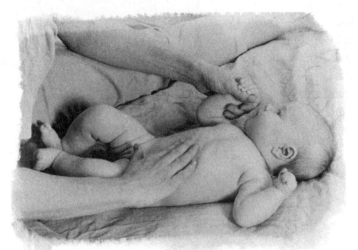

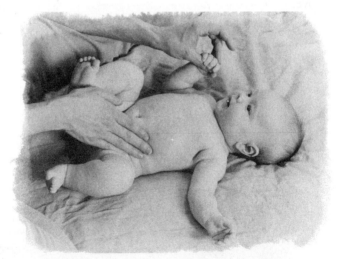

7. WALKING. Using the flat part of your fingers, walk across the baby's tummy at the navel, from your left to right. You may feel some gas bubbles moving under your fingers. After massaging the tummy, we move smoothly into the chest strokes.

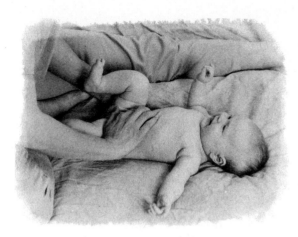

"May I Massage Your Chest?"

Massaging the chest helps tone the lungs and the heart. Imagine that you are freeing the baby's breath, and filling her heart with love. Begin by greeting the baby's chest with Resting Hands.

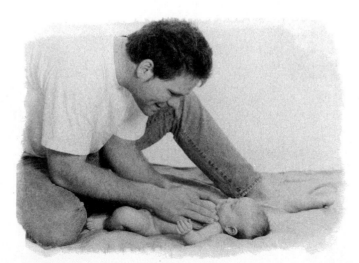

1. OPEN BOOK. With both hands together at the center of the chest, stroke out to the sides, following the rib cage, as if you were flattening the pages of a book. Keep your hands in contact with your baby as you move them down, around, and up to your starting point again, similar to a heart-shaped motion. The pressure is from the center of the chest outward; the rest is just to keep hands in contact with the body.

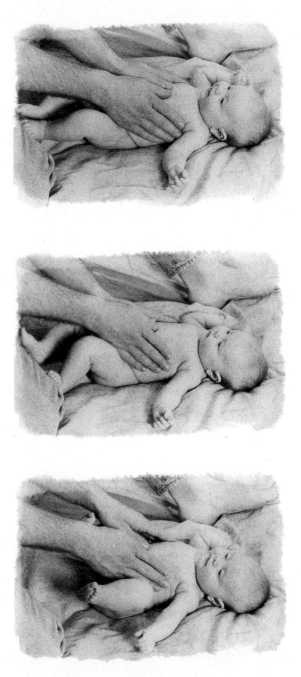

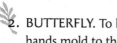

2. BUTTERFLY. To begin this stroke, both hands mold to the baby's rib cage.

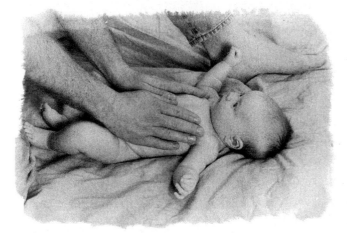

The right hand moves across the chest diagonally, to the baby's right shoulder. Then, pulling gently at the shoulder, the hand moves back diagonally to the rib cage. Be careful not to nick the baby's chin with your fingernails.

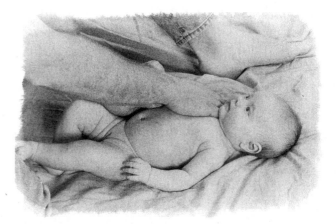

Now the left hand moves across the chest diagonally, to the baby's left shoulder, repeating the
same motion. Follow one hand with the other,
rhythmically crisscrossing the chest. There is more
pressure on the forward motion than coming back.
Remember to move from your center of gravity—
your lower back—keeping your arms and hands
relaxed and warm.

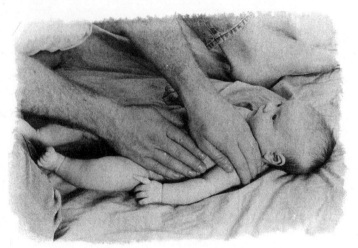

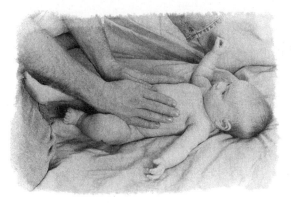

3. INTEGRATION.
Sweep both
hands from
chest, to tummy,
all the way to the
feet, to integrate
all of the strokes
you have just
performed.

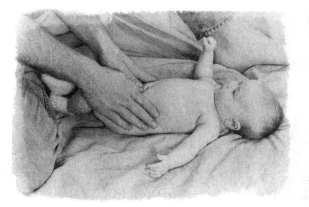

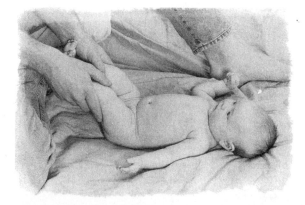

"May I Massage Your Arms and Hands?"

When massaging the arms, the complementary differences between Swedish and Indian methods are strikingly revealed in the Milking motions.

The traditional Indian way is to "milk" the arm from shoulder to wrist, imagining stress and tension leaving the body through the fingertips. The Swedish method is just the opposite, milking from wrist to shoulder, toward the heart. We use both methods, combining the Indian concept of balancing and releasing energy with the muscle-toning Swedish massage to promote good circulation.

1. RESTING HANDS. Start by greeting your baby's arms with warm, gentle touch and requesting permission.

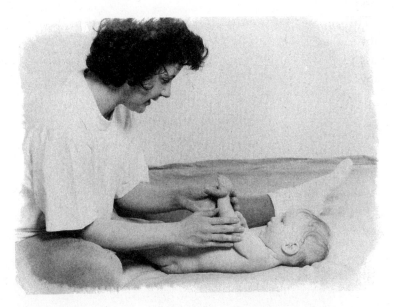

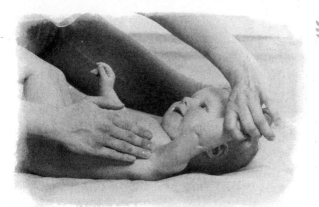

2. PIT STOP.
First stroke the armpit a few times, massaging the important lymph nodes in that area.

Some babies resist having their arms massaged and will protectively hug their arms close to their chest. In this case, rather than pulling outward on your baby's arm, massage it toward the direction she is holding it. Support her in protecting herself, massaging the arm in its "hug" position. When she begins to feel relaxed and supported, she will begin to relax her arms and "give" them to you for massage.

This photo shows the Indian Milking stroke being done with the baby holding her arm in tight. The parent supports her in that, just massaging in the way that she can in this position. Usually then the baby will begin to open up.

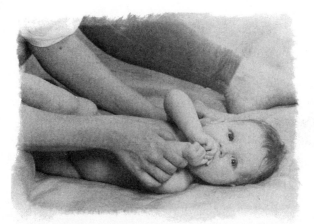

3. INDIAN MILKING. Holding your baby's wrist with your hand, milk the arm with the other hand, starting at the shoulder and moving to the wrist. Immediately follow with your other hand, and so forth, one hand after the other. Use the inside of your hand, molding your hand as much as possible to the baby's arm. Again, the inside edge of your hand, where your forefinger and thumb meet, should be facing you. For tiny babies, you may have to start just using three or four fingers; eventually, you can use your whole hand in a warm, encompassing stroke. Stabilize the baby's shoulder so as not to pull the body up off the surface.

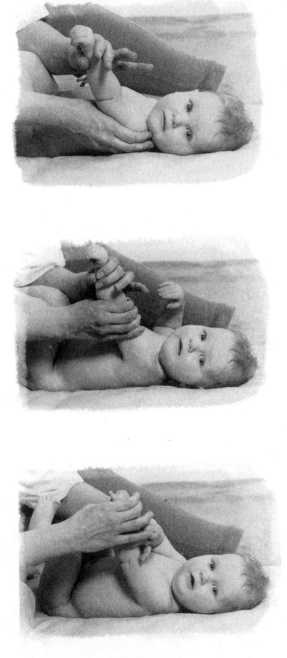

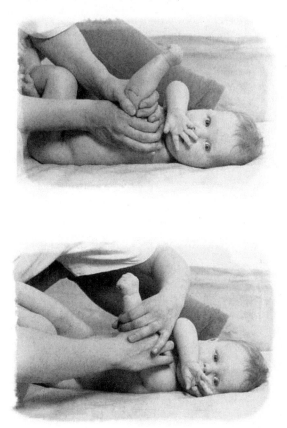

4. HUG AND GLIDE. Hold your hands together around the baby's arm, then very gently move your hands in opposite directions, keeping your hands together so as not to twist the elbow joint. With this stroke, you are gently massaging across the muscle, encouraging it to relax.

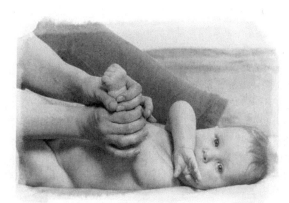

5. FINGER ROLL. Open your baby's hand with your thumbs, and roll each tiny finger between your index finger and thumb.

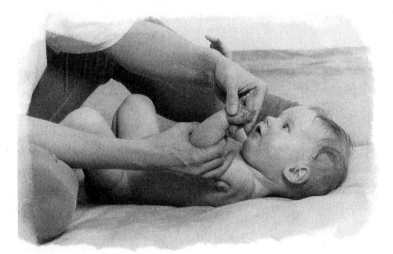

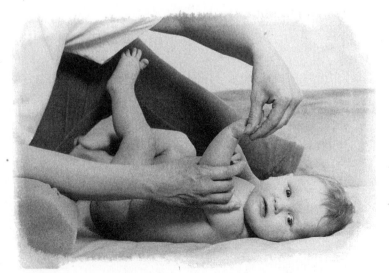

6. TOP OF HAND. Stroke the top of the hand.

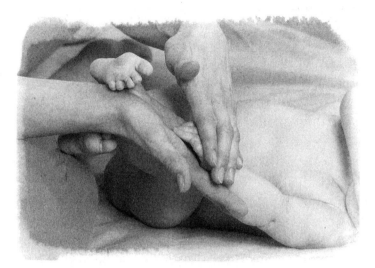

7. WRIST CIRCLES. Massage the wrist, making small circles all around.

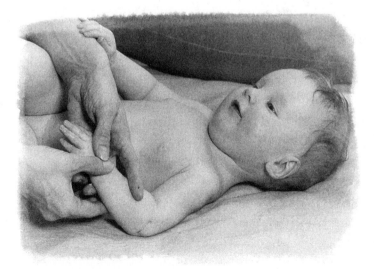

8. SWEDISH MILKING. Milk the arm from the wrist to the shoulder, one hand following another. Just as in Indian Milking (and with hands in the same position), try to mold your hand to the baby's arm. Stabilize your baby's shoulder so as not to pull the body up. Again, with tiny babies, you may use only three or four fingers to do this stroke at first.

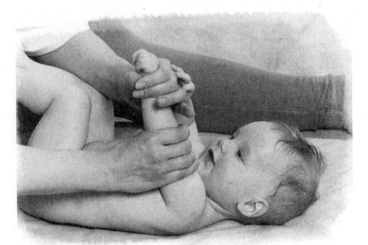

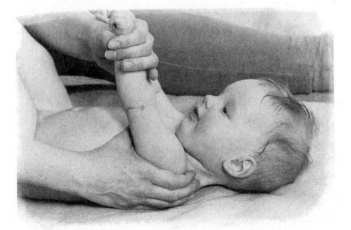

9. ROLLING. Roll your baby's arm between your hands from shoulder to wrist, several times. This is a fun stroke for babies of any age!

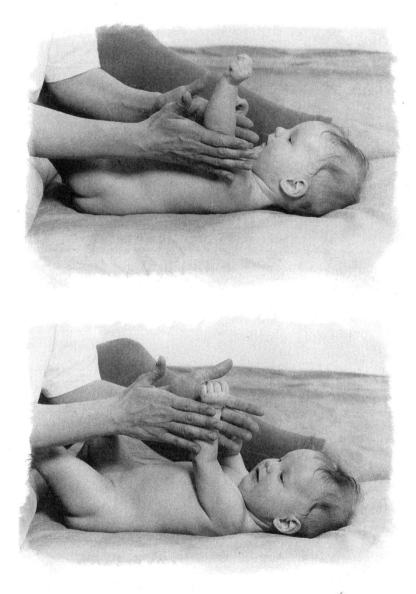

10. TOUCH RELAXATION. Use Touch Relaxation to help your baby relax and release her arm. Gently mold your hands to the baby's arm, letting your hands feel heavy and relaxed. Use your voice, saying, "Relax," or "Let go," as you gently pat, roll, and bounce the arm to encourage muscle relaxation. When you feel the muscles relax, give your baby good feedback: "Very good! You relaxed your arm!"

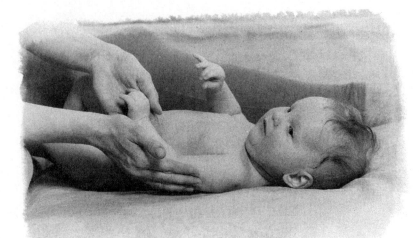

11. **INTEGRATION.** Sweep your hands from baby's shoulders, to chest, to tummy, to legs, to feet, in a single stroke integrating the whole body.

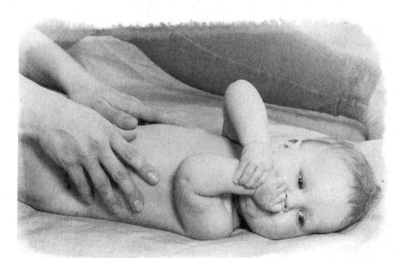

"May I Massage Your Face?"

A baby's face accumulates a lot of tension by sucking, teething, crying, and generally interacting with the world around her. I am often asked why I do not include strokes for the head here, and focus instead on the face. There are several reasons why. First, many infants' heads are sensitive, their bones still moving and growing as the plates shift and the soft spot hardens. Second, massaging the head can cause memories of the difficulty of pushing out of the birth canal, and so birth-trauma–type crying can ensue. In addition, there is no real musculature in the head that needs relaxing at this point. When your baby is four to six months old and you are very familiar with the massage, try cupping baby's head and making small circles, to see if she likes it or not. If so, you can include it in your routine at this point.

1. OPEN BOOK. Using the flat part of your fingers, start at the middle of the forehead and stroke out to the sides, as if flattening the pages of a book, moving your hands down along the sides of the face. Try not to cover your baby's eyes and nose with your hands.

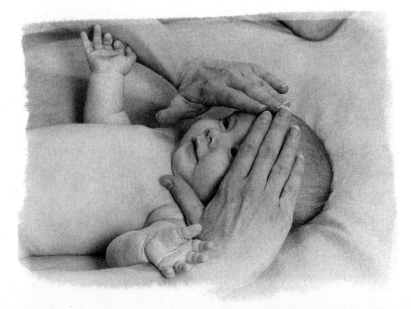

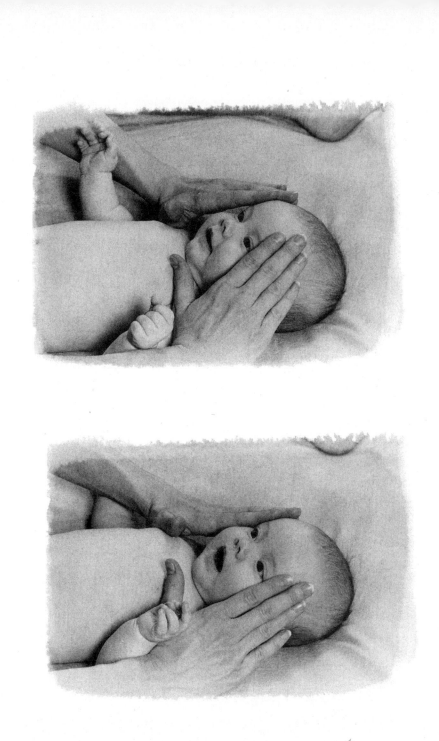

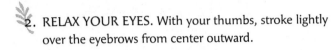

2. RELAX YOUR EYES. With your thumbs, stroke lightly over the eyebrows from center outward.

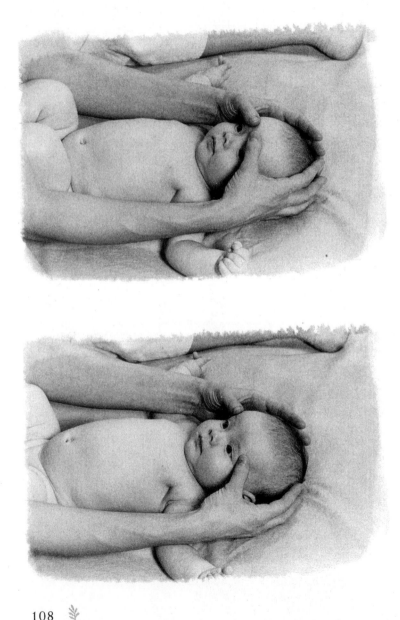

3. HAPPY SINUSES AND CHEEK MUSCLES. With your thumbs, push up on the bridge of the baby's nose, then stroke down diagonally across the cheeks. This helps open the sinuses and relax the cheek muscles.

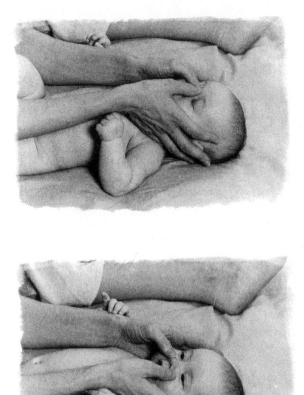

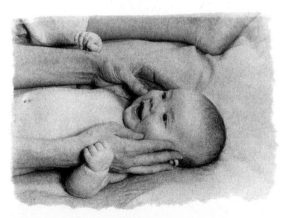

4. SMILE. With your thumbs, make a smile on
the upper, then the lower lip.

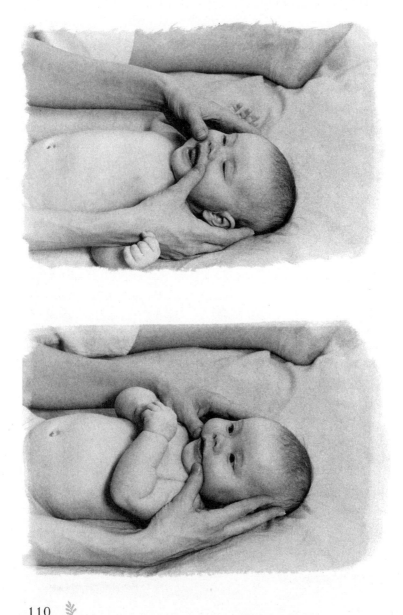

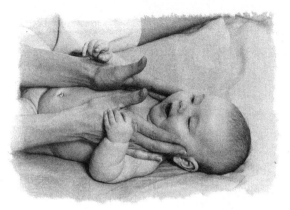

5. RELAX THE JAW. Make small circles around the jaw with your fingertips.

6. EARS, NECK, AND ALL OF THOSE CHINS! Using the fingertips of both hands, stroke over the ears, around the back of the ears, and pull up under the chin. This helps relax the jaw and massages the lymph nodes in this area. After these facial strokes, turn your baby over on her tummy for the back massage.

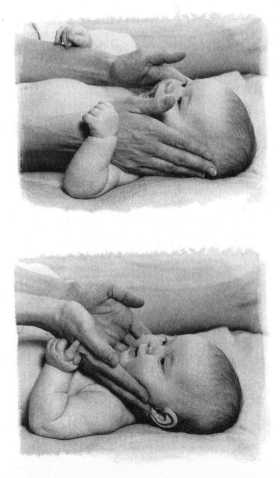

"May I Massage Your Back?"

The back is often a favorite with babies and toddlers alike. It can be the most relaxing part of the massage. These strokes also act as a warm-up for the gentle exercises that follow. To massage the back, turn your baby on his tummy, either on the table surface or on your lap with your legs extended. Older babies might like a toy to play with or a safe mirror to look at while the back is massaged.

1. RESTING HANDS. Position your baby and begin by relaxing yourself and letting the baby know the back massage is about to begin.

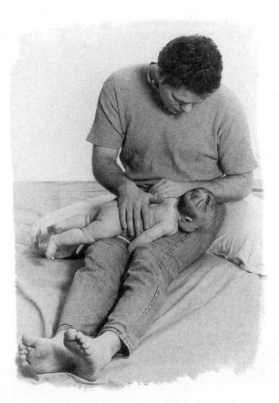

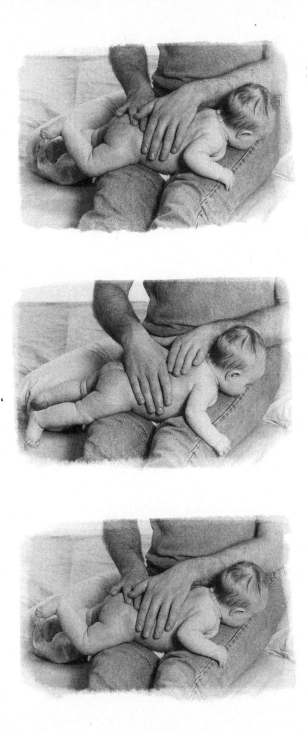

2. BACK AND FORTH. Start with both hands together at the top of the back, at right angles to the spine. Stroke your hands back and forth, perpendicular to the spine, alternating, molding your hands to the baby's back. Move down to the buttocks, then back up to the shoulders, and back down once again.

3. SWOOPING

PART A.
Keep one hand stationary at the buttocks. Then, beginning at the shoulders, the other hand swoops down to meet the hand at the buttocks. Mold your hand to the baby's back. Repeat this stroke several times.

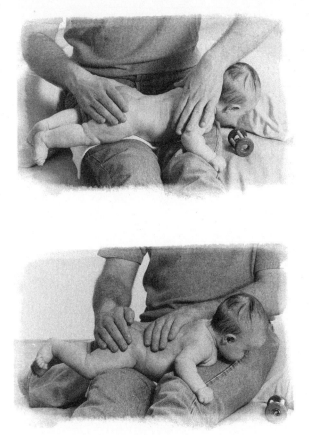

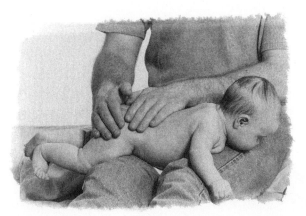

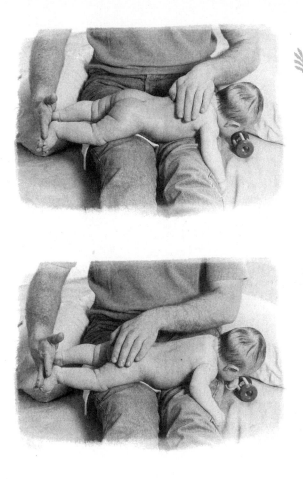

4. SWOOPING PART B. Holding one hand at your baby's feet (you may have to gently hold the feet still), swoop the other hand all the way down the back and the legs, to the ankles. Repeat several times.

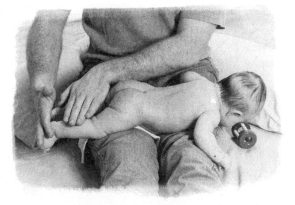

5. BACK CIRCLES. Make small circles all around the back with your fingertips. As your baby grows, you can feel muscles develop right under your fingertips!

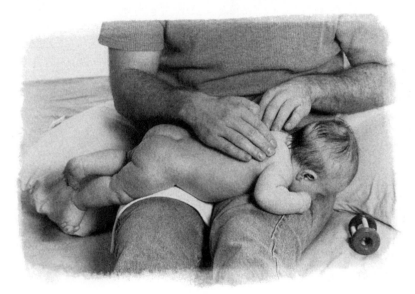

6. COMBING.
To finish the back, make "combing" strokes from the shoulders to buttocks, with your fingers spread apart, each stroke getting lighter and lighter, ending with a "feather touch." This tells your baby you are finished with the back.

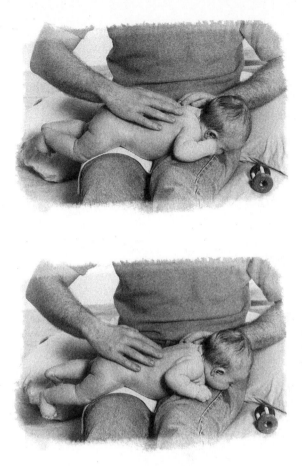

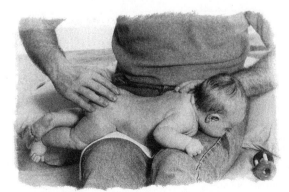

GENTLE MOVEMENTS

These movements are simple exercises that gently stretch baby's arms and legs, massage her stomach and pelvis, and align her spine. They are like yoga poses adapted for a baby. Be very gentle, and have fun with this routine, incorporating rhymes and games (see Chapter 13). After your baby begins to walk, these exercises will be unnecessary, as she will get plenty of stretching and exercise in day-to-day life.

1. CROSS ARMS. Cross your baby's arms at the chest three times, alternating which arm is over and under. Then gently stretch the arms out to the sides. The rhythm is: cross-cross-cross-open. Repeat.

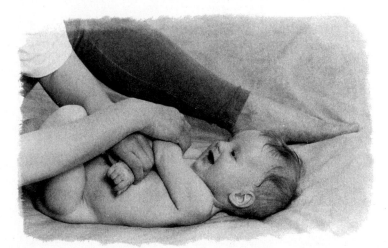

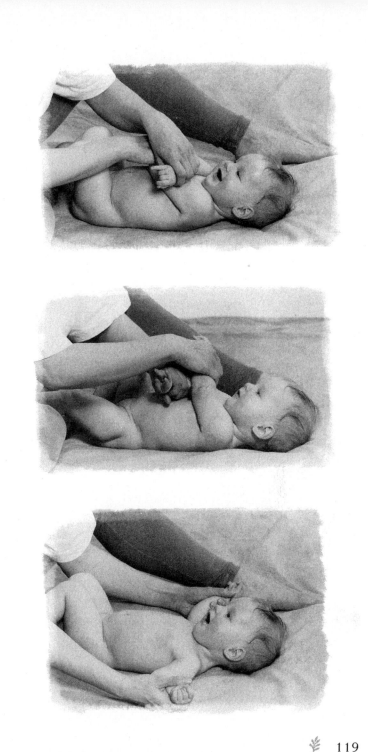

2. CROSS ARM AND LEG. Hold one arm at the wrist and the opposite leg at the ankle. Gently bring the arm down to the rib cage and the foot up toward the shoulder (allowing the knee to bend), then cross the leg and arm so that the arm goes to the outside of the leg, and cross again so the arm is under the leg, then cross once more with the arm over the leg. Now stretch them out in opposite directions. The rhythm is: cross-cross-cross-open. Repeat with the opposite arm and leg. Note: With an older baby, bring the knee, rather than the foot, up to cross with the arm.

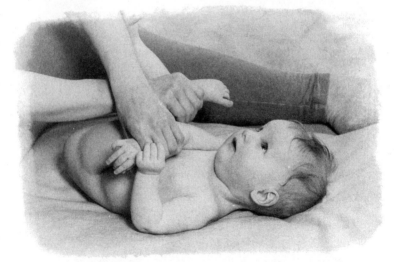

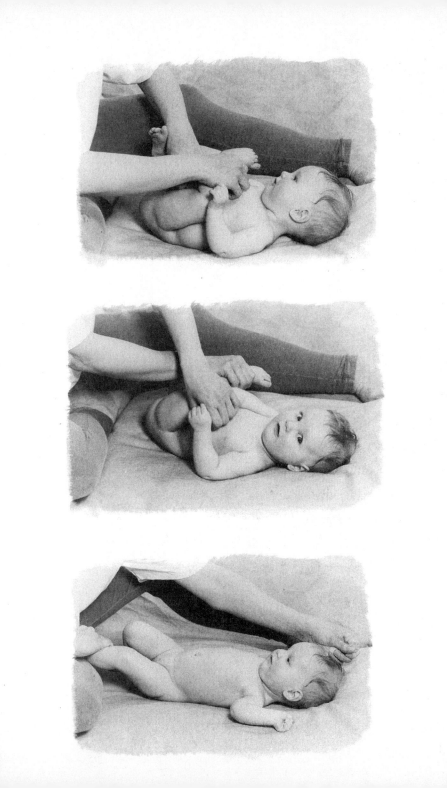

3. CROSS LEGS. Cross the legs over the tummy three times, alternating which leg is over and under. Then gently stretch the legs out straight, toward you. The rhythm is cross-cross-cross-straighten. Repeat. This is a good exercise for toning the digestive tract.

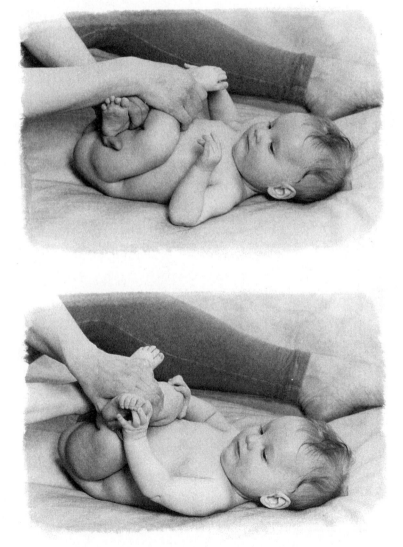

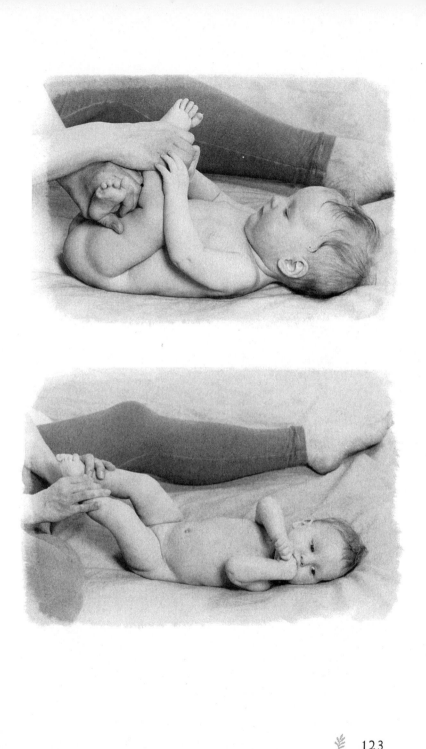

4. UP DOWN. Push the knees together up into the tummy, then stretch them out straight. If the baby resists straightening her legs, bounce them gently and encourage her to relax. Repeat several times.

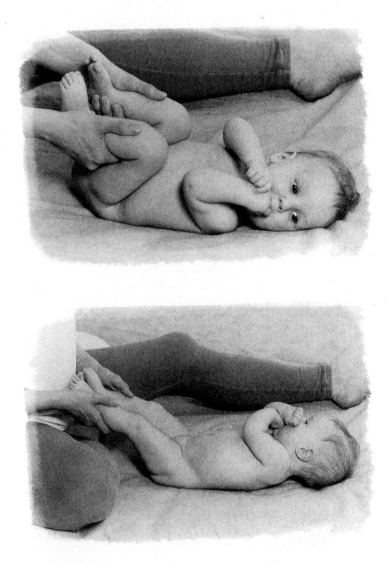

5. BICYCLE.
Gently push
the knees into
the tummy,
one after the
other, then
bounce them
out straight
to relax.
The rhythm is
push right—
push left—
push right—
straighten,
alternating the
leg you start
with each
time.

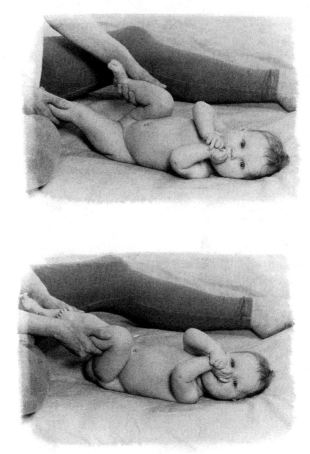

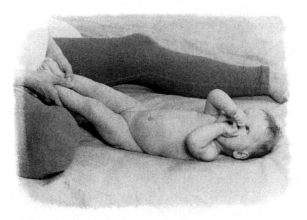

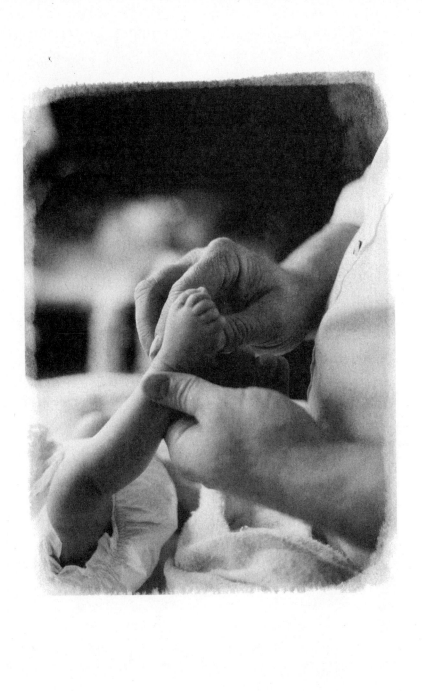

Abbreviated Massage

Sometimes you want to give your baby a quick rubdown on the run, when changing his diaper or just before bed. Here is an abbreviated massage that will take only a few minutes but will still provide the benefits of communication and relaxation your baby needs. This massage can be done with or without oil or lotion.

1. Cup head in hands. If baby likes, make circles around head.

2. Open Book, on forehead

3. Relax the Jaw

4. Open Book, on chest

5. Rolling, on arms; open hands

6. Sun Moon or I Love You, on stomach

7. Rolling, on legs

8. Thumb Press, on soles of feet

9. Back and Forth, on back

10. Combing, on back

REVIEW OF THE STROKES

1. Relax and breathe deeply as you remove your jewelry and your baby's clothing, covering the genitals with a cloth or diaper.

2. Oil your palms, and rub them together to warm them up.

3. Show your palms to your baby and request permission to begin.

4. Legs and Feet:
   a. Resting Hands
   b. Indian Milking
   c. Hug and Glide
   d. Thumb over Thumb
   e. Toe Roll
   f. Under Toes
   g. Heel of Foot
   h. Thumb Press
   i. Top of Foot
   j. Ankle Circles
   k. Swedish Milking
   l. Rolling
   m. Bottom Relaxer
   n. Integration

5. Stomach:
   a. Resting Hands
   b. Water Wheel Part A and Part B
   c. Thumbs to Sides
   d. Sun Moon
   e. I Love You
   f. Walking

6. Chest
   a. Resting Hands
   b. Open Book
   c. Butterfly
   d. Integration

7. Arms and Hands
   a. Resting Hands
   b. Pit Stop
   c. Indian Milking
   d. Hug and Glide
   e. Open Hand and Finger Roll
   f. Top of Hand
   g. Wrist Circles
   h. Swedish Milking
   i. Rolling
   j. Touch Relaxation
   k. Integration

8. Face
   a. Open Book
   b. Relax Your Eyes
   c. Happy Sinuses and Cheek Muscles
   d. Smile
   e. Relax the Jaw
   f. Ears, Neck, and All of Those Chins!

9. Back
   a. Resting Hands
   b. Back and Forth
   c. Swooping Part A and Part B
   d. Back Circles
   e. Combing

10. Gentle Movements
    a. Cross Arms
    b. Cross Arm and Leg
    c. Cross Legs
    d. Up Down
    e. Bicycle

11. *And a kiss to grow on!*

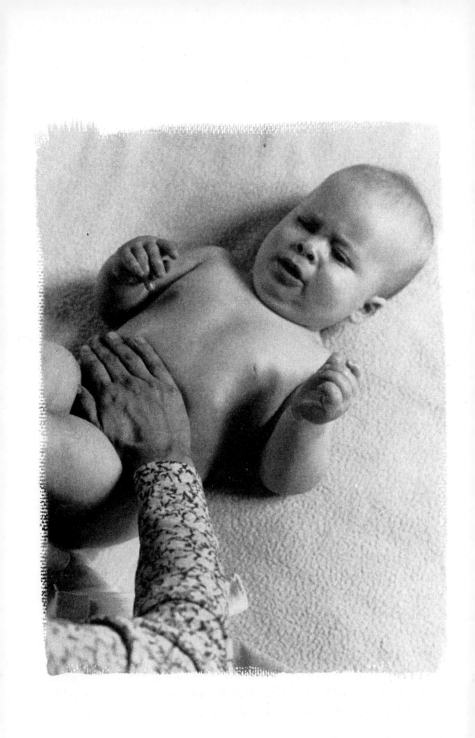

Chapter 9

Crying, Fussing, and Other Baby Language

This is my sad time of day.
—Arnold Lobel

A T THIS POINT, you may be imagining yourself lovingly massaging your baby as he lies there contentedly listening to your voice, gazing into your eyes, and perhaps even falling asleep. This will probably happen quite often, and when it does, it is wonderful. But most babies will fuss or cry at times during a massage. If you understand the reasons for your baby's fussiness, you will be much more comfortable and better able to help him.

Because infants grow so rapidly, there is often much tension in their little bodies. They work so hard to develop muscle coordination that occasionally they may well ache and feel out of sorts.

When your body aches, a massage feels both good and uncomfortable at the same time. Your muscles are sore, and even a gentle touch can bring discomfort. Still, being touched is so relaxing, and getting blood circulating through your sore muscles is so healing, that your grunts and grimaces may mean either pain or pleasure. Often a massage can remind you of aches you never knew you had, but afterward the feelings of relief and release you experience are well worth it.

Massage is a new experience for your little one. At first she may react negatively to the sensations she experiences, but after she becomes accustomed to being touched in this fashion, she will begin to enjoy the routine. So take it easy at first, and acquaint her with these new sensations slowly. You, too, may feel clumsy and flustered at first, trying to learn the strokes and do them "correctly," leading to tension on your part, which your baby will pick up.

Babies who had a difficult or traumatic birth, who had difficulties afterward for which they needed medical intervention, or who have just come from foster homes or orphanages, tend to have more negative reactions to being massaged at first. For example, babies who have received routine heel sticks for blood testing often cry when their feet are massaged, even several months later. If your baby seems to be reacting negatively to particular parts of the massage, use Touch Relaxation techniques and gentle Resting Hands first, gradually introducing massage strokes as they are accepted.

CARRYING

Some babies just need a lot of in-arms time, and the vast array of front packs and slings now available make it easier for both parents to respond to a baby's need for closeness. In one study, mothers of newborns were divided into two groups: one group was given plastic infant seats, the other soft baby carrier packs. At three months, the babies who had been carried often in the soft carriers looked more often at their mothers and cried less than those who had spent most of their time in the infant seats. At thirteen months, the carried babies were more likely to be securely attached to their parents than the infant seat group. Lately, Kangaroo Care has been in fashion in hospitals for medically fragile and/or premature infants.

But full-term, healthy babies seem to benefit tremendously from being carried a lot, too. Maybe those mothers in "primitive" tribes who carry their infants in slings and packs are on to something!

Carrying an infant in a pack also provides the benefits of stimulating the baby's gastrointestinal system, slowing the heart rate, promoting more effective respiratory functioning, and decreasing congestion. Moreover, the familiar rhythms and rocking of a parent's body going about his or her daily activities are soothing and calming. As Terry Levy and Michael Orlans note in their book *Attachment, Trauma, and Healing*, "Infants who are placed in heart-to-heart proximity with a primary caregiver maintain a mutual heart synchrony."

In addition, carrier packs soothe babies by allowing them to stay warm and feel, as well as listen to, their parent's heartbeat. Heartbeat sounds have been shown to increase appetite and thus weight gain, to regulate sleep and respiration, and to reduce crying by fifty percent.

BABY'S CUES

Your baby has a lot to say but has not yet developed language. So he uses his body language, cries, coos, and other sounds to communicate with you. Pay close attention to these signals. Your baby is teaching you his unique way of saying what he wants you to hear. Dr. Linda Acredolo and Dr. Susan Goodwyn, authors of *Baby Signs: How to Talk with Your Baby Before Your Baby Can Talk*, recognized this tendency in babies to "sign" before learning speech. In their fascinating book, they show how babies make up signs for objects and feelings and teach them to their parents. The parents, if they are conscious of them, can then use the signs with their babies and attach words to them, so when a baby is ready to speak, the word comes easily. Later on, parents can also teach their babies signs for things, showing a sign and attaching a word to it, to help the baby develop language before speech. For example, a one-year-old may open and close her hands to indicate "book."

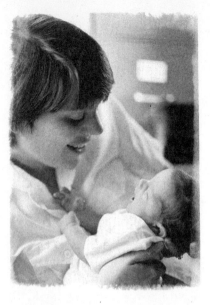

This way of "talking" before speech can be important to us in our babies' massage routine. Your palms swishing together can come to mean "massage," and asking your baby's permission further indicates that a massage is being offered. Often when a baby is feeling stressed out by the stimulation, she will give a sign or cue to let you know she needs a break. She may, for example, hold a hand up in front of her face as if to say "stop!" Sometimes hiccuping is a stress cue. If she looks around rapidly while fussing, she may need to be swaddled and comforted and/or rhythmically rocked or bounced (see "Fussing," later in this chapter) to bring her energies back into alignment and calm her.

I encourage you to begin teaching your baby signs for "massage," "no," "relax" (perhaps wiggling limp hands while saying the word "relax"); signs for the various body parts; signs for "happy," "sad," and "angry"; and a sign for "all done," even before the baby is capable of giving the signs back to you. Acredolo and Goodwyn say that Baby Signs will usually not be used until a baby is about nine months old at the earliest. But other researchers have found that even in the premature nursery, babies give "cues" to alert their caregivers of their state and their needs. You will learn your own baby's unique cues as you massage him day by day. Not all babies mean the same thing when they hiccup, hold up a hand, or look away. Allow your baby to teach you what he means by the various signs he gives you through his body language. Often during a massage, a baby will go through a very short period of stress-release fussing, in which he gives these stress cues but then settles down and enjoys the rest of the massage. The idea is simply to be aware of your baby's unique expressions and to help her give words to her gestures so that when she is ready to talk, she knows exactly what to say.

STAGES OF GROWTH

Babies commonly react to the various massage strokes differently, according to their age and stage of development. But although every baby is unique, knowing the most common reactions to massage can help you adjust your strokes when and if your own baby displays them. Remember that during developmental growth spurts, babies can often become fussy and irritable. A warm, loving massage can help them release the tension that this rapid growth can cause.

During the first three months of life, your baby displays many neonatal reflexes. The tonic neck reflex causes his head to turn to the side; the moro reflex causes him to startle when his head is unsupported. Massaging your baby in a "cradle" of sorts will offer him warmth and support and keep his head aligned if he wants to make eye contact with you. Many newborns hold their arms in tightly, with their fists closed, and they become anxious when their arms are massaged. If your baby does this to an extreme, use Touch Relaxation to help him relax and release this tension before you introduce the massage strokes. Observe your baby closely, and you will see how hard he works to strengthen and coordinate his arms. Because he held them near his body for months in the womb, having them pulled away may feel downright scary. In addition, the arms may be programmed biologically to protect the vital organs in the chest area. Show him it is okay to open and relax his arms. In the beginning, arms are also exercised by "push-ups"—the baby's attempts to look up when placed on his belly. Touch his arms in a gentle and loving way, and stroke with, rather than against, the way he naturally holds them. He will probably enjoy the strokes for the legs and back during this period, and this feeling will, in turn, help him to relax his arms.

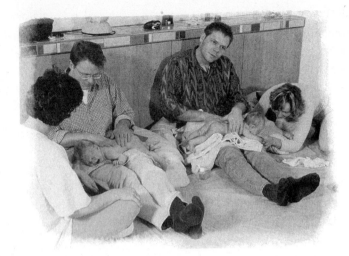

During the second three months of life, most babies begin to look around their environment and enjoy interacting with people. Your baby will begin to learn how to roll over during this stage; if he wants to do so during the massage, let him, and simply adjust the massage routine, stroking his back and legs. Tension appears in the back, too, because the baby is exercising these muscles in preparation for crawling and standing. The face may also hold tension from crying, teething, sucking, and interacting so intensely with people. At this stage, many babies particularly enjoy having their stomachs, chests, and arms massaged.

For seven-to-twelve-month-old babies, mobility is a major focus. Massage is a challenge for such babies because they are so intent upon moving about: massage is less a relaxing experience than a playtime activity or a bedtime ritual. You can invent strokes that are useful as your baby moves around, making a game of getting a massage. Songs, rhymes, finger-plays, and stories can help you keep the baby's attention at this age.

Toward the end of the first year, tension may move into the baby's legs as she learns to stand and walk. This can be an especially trying time, and some babies will steadfastly refuse to be massaged at all. Every bit of her attention may be focused on walking and teething. She may be very fussy and short-tempered until she's mastered the art of walking and has most of their teeth. Then she will slow down a little, having accomplished these gargantuan feats. In Chapter 13, we will explore in further detail how to change the massage routine as your child grows older.

FUSSING

Some babies need time to become accustomed to being massaged and will, at first, become fussy after just a few minutes. Breathe deeply, and make every effort to relax yourself. Then allow the baby to fuss a little. Often he will release the tension during the massage, and the massage itself will make him a lot happier, more relaxed, and able to sleep more soundly. As tension is released and the baby's stimulation threshold rises, the fussing will diminish.

If your baby consistently begins to fuss at a certain point in the massage, it may be that he needs a break or a shorter massage period for a while. You can take a break to nurse or cuddle, then try again. If he continues to fuss, you may try massaging for a shorter period, at a different time of day, starting on a different area of the body. Check to be sure he is warm enough and that you are relaxed and comfortable. Listen closely to what he says with his fussing; perhaps he needs to tell you about his day! Check for gas or colic (Chapter 10), and listen, listen, listen. Your baby has a lot to say and needs to be heard.

When Your Baby Is "Disorganized"

Sometimes your baby will fuss because he feels overstimulated, stressed out, tired, and unable to gather his energies back together and either rest or go to sleep. Mothers worldwide have invented many techniques to help babies when they feel "disorganized." Holding her in the manner she likes while rocking or walking her can help. Sometimes a warm bath can help. Some parents even drive the baby around in the car!

The technique I saw done most often in India was one I found to be useful with my babies and many of the babies in my classes. I call it Indian Bouncing. It is very simple.

INDIAN BOUNCING. You lay your baby across your lap, face down, making sure he has room to breathe, parting your legs a bit for his tummy. Be sure your baby's head is supported to prevent harming his delicate neck; let the baby's cheek or chin rest on a folded blanket or towel on your legs. Never let baby's head hang off your leg. Then lay warm, relaxed Resting Hands on his back. Now, very gently bounce your knees up and down rhythmically and *slowly,* as you gently pat your baby's back at the same rate with slightly cupped hands.

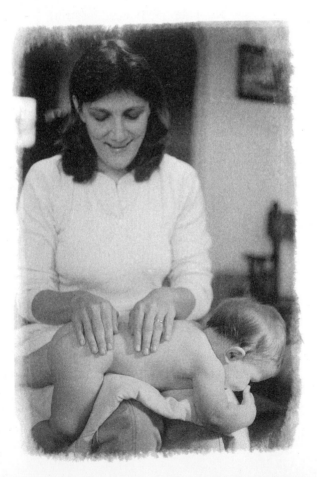

Do this rhythmic bouncing for about five minutes. Usually the baby will either fall asleep or stop fussing and relax into the rhythm. If and when he feels centered again, you may put him down for a nap or carry on with your day. When I traveled by train in India, I often observed mothers in groups with their babies across their knees, patting and bouncing them as they talked to one another. Everyone seemed to be having a wonderful time! In the orphanage where I worked and in Mother Teresa's baby hospital, this method was also used, with swaddling, to help a baby or toddler whose energies seemed "out of control."

CRYING

Once I was asked to demonstrate infant massage for a television news spot. As the host and I hurried to the studio, she said, "I hear you have a way to stop a baby's screams in ten seconds flat with massage. I hope you can show us that today!"

The baby, a sweet four-month-old with whom I'd had a lovely conversation in the waiting room, took one look at the newscaster and began to cry inconsolably. I did not demonstrate massage on her, because I felt that using massage as a trick to quiet her (even if it worked, which I doubt) would betray her feelings and her body. The host concluded that the infant massage gimmick did not work. She was right. As a gimmick, it does not. Unfortunately, many people think that babies should be seen and not heard.

As infants, we had few ways beyond crying to express our negative feelings and release pent-up stress. While growing up, we learned to deal with anger, fear, pain, and excess energy in many ways; our facial expressions, body language, and speech patterns now help us to convey how we feel. When the stresses of living pile up, we can go for a walk, take a vacation, or talk to a friend. We cry from time to time, even when we are healthy, but rarely in front of others. We have learned that crying is antisocial and a sign of weakness. This was probably one of our earliest lessons.

Do Babies Manipulate Parents with Crying?

The injunction not to "spoil" a baby came into vogue in the early part of the twentieth century. People began to think that they should let a crying baby "cry it out" alone. The rationale was that babies used crying to manipulate parents into gratifying their desires, and that this was an unattractive character trait. Responding to crying could only cultivate spoiled, boorish children who would lead their parents around by the nose. In order to prevent babies from manipulating and to train them for independence early, parents left them alone to cry until they grew hoarse and fell asleep from sheer exhaustion. But the validity of this approach has been disproven again and again. Infants' needs are real, and they cry for real reasons. They do not have the intellectual sophistication to manipulate their parents.

In the 1970s, a movement away from this earlier practice gained momentum. Many more women began breastfeeding; front- and backpacks and folding "umbrella" strollers were invented; and baby experts encouraged parents to interact more closely with and respond more quickly to their infants. Research told us that babies who are responded to cry less, not more, and are more rather than less independent later on. Other cultures have further influenced this change. As global communications have become more sophisticated, they have allowed Westerners to look more closely at cultures that have not yet been impaired by so-called modern thinking.

Unfortunately, we in the West have been so impaired. Mothers who previously might have left their baby alone to cry while they felt guilty and tearful in the adjacent room now jumped at the baby's smallest peep. But something remained: getting the baby to stop crying, or not allowing the baby to cry at all, was still our obsession.

Today, in many people's minds, the pendulum has swung back to the thinking that babies become spoiled by being attended to and that they should be trained or "managed" to act according to what is convenient for their parents. It seems regardless of where we are on this continuum, we continually miss the point regarding a baby's need to cry.

At times, we all need to cry. It is a release, and crying in the loving arms of another person is often much more so. I believe that babies' feelings are as deep as ours, that their fears, their sorrows, and their frustrations are no less. From observing hundreds of babies in massage classes and in other cultures, I know that crying can sometimes be a relief and a release for infants.

Many of us brought up in the age of "don't spoil the baby" have mixed feelings about crying. We get anxious, tense up, and want the crying to stop right away. Crying triggers our fears and perhaps reminds us of the anguish, fear, and anger we may have felt crying alone in a crib with no response. It can also engender guilt: Am I a bad mother if my baby cries?

Our culture often reinforces negative feelings about crying. Many people become extremely agitated by any noise a baby makes and assail the parents with dour looks at the slightest sound. The embarrassed parent often responds by punishing the baby with loud hisses, apologizing for the baby, and fleeing for the safety of home. Because of our society's lack of support for childrearing, the demands of our economy, and social values that do not encourage family bonding, most new parents periodically experience extremely high levels of stress, regardless of their parenting philosophies. Who among us has not thought of "throwing the baby out the window" or feared losing control and shaking or yelling at a crying baby? When you are overwhelmed by these feelings, if possible ask your partner to hold the baby while you remove yourself to a quiet place for five or ten minutes to practice Controlled Belly Breathing and release your anxiety. If you feel so frustrated that you want to cry, go ahead. When my children were babies, we sometimes paced the living room together, both mother and baby crying through our pain and frustration. We should begin to accept crying as simply another way we humans can cleanse our hearts of negative feelings and stress. We can acknowledge that it is okay to cry sometimes, and that everyone eventually

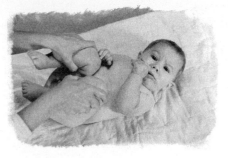

stops crying and finds relief, especially if their family and friends allow them to express their feelings, and love and respect them all the more for doing so.

Like all of us, babies have many different reasons for crying. Unfortunately, we have lost much of our capacity to intuit their thoughts and feelings. Most people are able to recognize a sharp cry of pain, but our interpretations of other cries and fusses are filtered through the veil of our own insecurities and projections. It may be easier to adopt a mechanistic philosophy that sees all crying as alike, to be responded to in the same way—either by ignoring or by hushing. But babies are not interested in philosophy, and they are unable to attend to their parents' comfort. They need clear-thinking, caring, centered adults to help them find their way through this world of unknowns. Daily massage can help you learn to understand your baby's vocalizations intuitively because it helps you to literally keep in touch with your baby's body language, nonverbal signals, and different types of cries.

Actively and compassionately listening to an infant isn't much different from listening to a child or adult. It requires empathy, genuine love, and respect for the person's experience. The reason it is so difficult for us to listen to our babies, I believe, is that our own infancies may have been full of frustration and unheard feelings. When we hear our babies cry, rather than truly listening to what they are saying, we superimpose our own inner infant. Our overwhelming impulse is to quiet *that* baby. We hush our babies as we ourselves were hushed.

Research has consistently shown that babies who are responded to promptly—not by hushing but by listening and acting—cry less frequently and for shorter periods as they grow older. Crying releases hormones that reduce tension and arousal. It is not only an expression of pain or discomfort but seems to be an inborn stress-management and healing mechanism. If allowed and responded to with relaxed, loving listening, crying can help babies regulate their own stress levels and grow to be more relaxed and stress-free children and adults.

HOW TO LISTEN TO A BABY

When your baby begins to vocalize, fuss, or cry during massage, you can use a three-step process. First, take a long, slow, deep breath, and relax your whole body. This directly counteracts the tendency to hold your breath and tighten up.

Second, set aside your own inner infant for a moment. In order to truly hear your baby, you must clear yourself and realize that your baby has his own reasons for crying. Third, make eye contact with your baby if possible. If he is avoiding eye contact, place your hands gently but firmly on his body, and connect with him through your hands. Let your love go to him, telling him with your voice, your eyes, and your hands that you would like to hear what he has to say.

Stay with the baby, keeping yourself very relaxed and receptive. Listen and respond to him, observing his body language. Watch his mouth and what he says with his eyes. When you are sure he feels heard and has said most of what he has to say, offer the comfort of rocking, walking, and cuddling to help him get organized again. Invariably, a baby who feels he has been heard will sleep more deeply afterward and will extend himself in trust more the next time.

When we truly listen to our infants, we are fulfilling all of their psychological needs. Our underlying message is "You are worthy of respect. You are valuable just the way you are." The baby takes in this message, and her whole body relaxes. The chalice of her heart is filled to overflowing, and as she grows, she will seek opportunities to share her love with others. How will she do this? By following the model she has been given. She will be there for others in the way you have been there for her. What a lovely, healthy cycle!

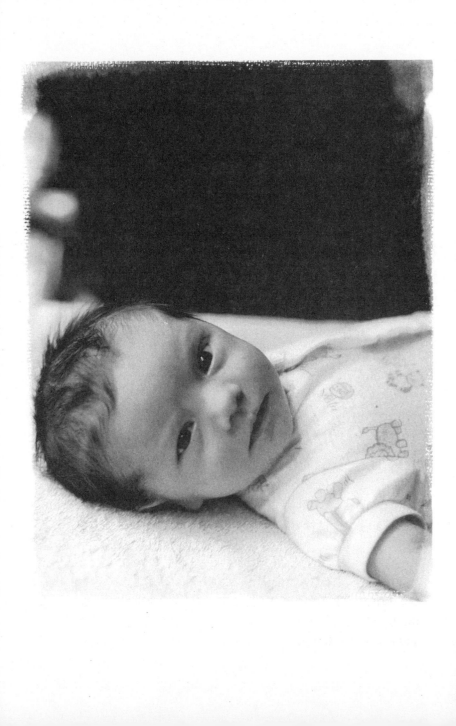

Chapter 10

Minor Illness and Colic

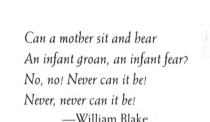

Can a mother sit and hear
An infant groan, an infant fear?
No, no! Never can it be!
Never, never can it be!
—William Blake

IN TIMES OF ILLNESS, a massage not only can comfort but can also help relieve painful symptoms such as aches, fever, congestion, and the labored breathing of croup and asthma. Of course, as with any significant deviation from health in your baby, consult your family doctor about its use.

FEVER

To help bring down a fever, use some of the same strokes as in the basic massage. Use warm water on your hands instead of oil, and except for the part you are working on, keep the baby's body covered. Working from the chest to the extremities, dip your hand in the water, then briskly rub the body. The idea is to bring the heat up to the surface of the skin, where the water will evaporate and help cool it. Whenever the baby has a fever, check with the physician. My own baby's pediatrician taught me this method as a way to bring down a fever when my baby had ear infections.

CHEST CONGESTON

You can use another technique to help ease chest congestion. First, do the regular massage strokes for the chest, using oil on your hands, adding a drop of eucalyptus or Mentholatum. Tip the baby at a slight angle, with his head down. Using a small cup (the clean plastic cup from the top of a cough syrup bottle works nicely) or something with a small rim, press in and pull out gently all over the chest and back. The gentle suction helps pull mucus away from the lungs so it can be coughed up. A vaporizer in the baby's room can help, too. Be sure the vaporizer is very clean so it is not putting harmful bacteria into the air. This method is useful for baby "croup" and asthma as well. Again, consult with the baby's pediatrician first.

NASAL CONGESTION

For nasal congestion, assemble the following: a nasal aspirator, a dropper, a handkerchief, and a cup of warm salted water (ratio: one-half teaspoon salt per cup of warm water). Do the massage strokes for the face, especially the ones for the sinus area, to help relax the area, increase circulation, and loosen mucus. Place a drop of the warm salted water in each nostril. Push the bulb end of the aspirator closed. Now, carefully and gently insert the aspirator tip into the baby's nostril. Release the pressure on the bulb, and suction out the mucus with the aspirator, blowing it into the handkerchief. The warm salt water is easy on her nose and will help loosen the mucus considerably. She will not enjoy this process, but it may be necessary if her stuffiness is preventing her from sucking, and it is better to avoid using over-the-counter medicines if possible. Her own antibodies will fight the cold and will be stronger next time in immunizing her against viruses. After you are finished, comfort the baby and feed her. Be sure you clean all of the items very carefully with boiling water, to kill any bacteria, before using them again.

GAS AND COLIC

Babies often cry because of painful gas or because they are tired and their energies are disorganized. Discomfort and outright pain from trapped gas are very common. Since babies' gastrointestinal systems are immature at birth, they need prompting to begin functioning the way they should. Massage can provide just the right type of stimulation.

There has been much speculation over the years concerning colic and its causes. The label "colic" is often used for any baby who cries often; I prefer to use it for babies who cry for extended periods of time and are obviously experiencing stomach pain. A truly colicky baby is stiff and tense, has a distended abdomen, and has difficulty tolerating stimulation. A baby with discomfort from gas that is not so severe cries often, pulls his legs up and seems to be in pain, and may expel gas in short bursts. Often the gassy baby can be comforted by walking or rhythmic rocking and holding, while the colicky baby may or may not be comforted during an episode.

For several years, I worked with a pediatric practice, specifically helping families with colicky babies. Overwhelmed by the crying, the sleepless nights, and the feelings of helplessness and incompetence, parents often said things like "My baby just doesn't like me" or "I'm just not a good parent. I can't calm him down." They were distanced from their babies instead of bonding with them. But when I could show the parents how the baby's gastrointestinal system works, and how the massage routine helps to relax the area and release painful gas, they began to understand they were doing nothing wrong as parents. I started by helping the parents to relax. Virtually every family I worked with had remarkable results within two weeks of practicing this routine every day.

When parents could do the routine and get a result—that is, the baby would release gas either during the session or soon thereafter and begin to sleep for longer periods and cry less—the parents felt much more competent and began to see their babies in a more positive light, and bond with them again.

Massage can help any baby, from mildly gassy to extremely colicky, by stimulating the gastrointestinal system to do its job. It helps release built-up stress, and the Touch Relaxation and Resting Hands techniques help the baby learn to relax.

COLIC RELIEF ROUTINE

First of all, try to relax yourself. A gassy or colicky baby is a challenge for any parent, and your stress overload can make you feel edgy and confused. Remember, you are not at fault for your baby's discomfort, but you can help him. Listen to his cries with respect for his feelings, and then get to work to help him manage his episodes.

Massage the baby twice a day for two weeks, using the techniques given here. I suggest that you do this routine instead of the normal massage. That means if you have a very colicky baby who needs two weeks of twice-a-day colic relief, don't do the regular massage until after that period. In this way, the baby won't associate all massage with the discomfort that may be experienced during the Colic Relief Routine.

As you do this routine, remember to count the strokes and hold the knees-up position. Then help the baby relax with Touch Relaxation, using your voice, your hands, and rhythmic rocking, patting, and light bouncing to help him loosen up. When doing the knees-up position, do not press in too hard, just firmly; you don't want to cut off your baby's breathing!

1. RESTING HANDS. Rest your hands on your baby's tummy, relaxing yourself completely, even if the baby is fussing and crying.

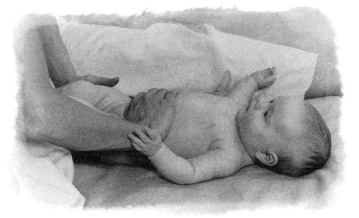

 2. WATER WHEEL PART A *(see page 85)*. Do this stroke six times, one hand following the other.

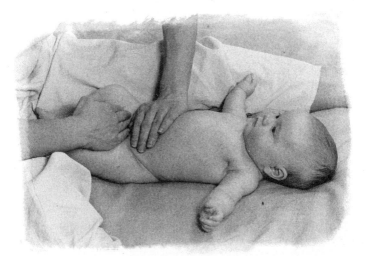

3. KNEES UP DOWN *(see page124)*. Hold the baby's knees together, then push gently up into his tummy, holding for about a half minute.

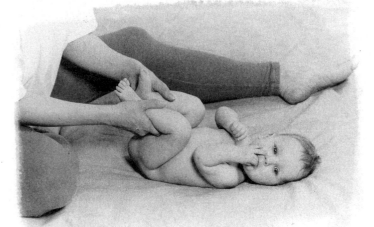

4. TOUCH RELAXATION. Gently release the pressure, stroke his legs, and use Touch Relaxation to coax him to release tension and relax.

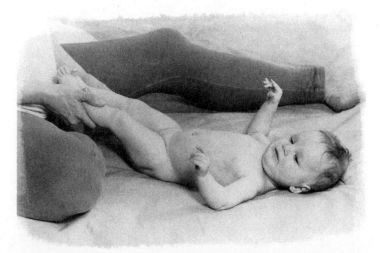

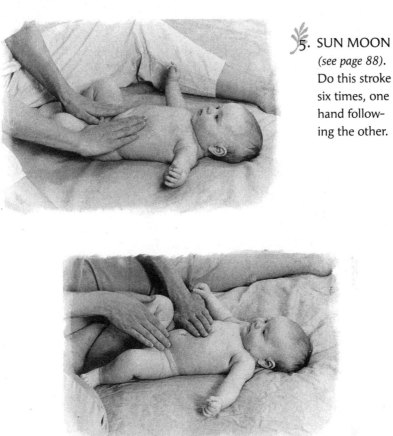

5. SUN MOON
(see page 88).
Do this stroke
six times, one
hand follow-
ing the other.

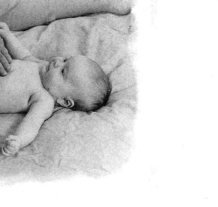

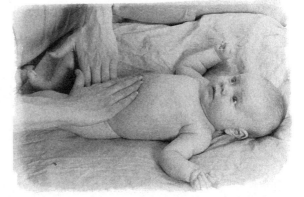

6. KNEES UP DOWN *(see page 124)*. Hold the baby's knees together and push gently up into his tummy, holding for about a half minute.

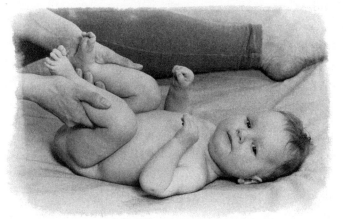

 7. TOUCH RELAXATION. Gently release the pressure, stroke his legs, and use Touch Relaxation to coax him to relax and release tension.

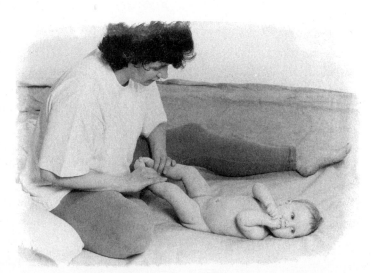

Repeat this entire cycle (steps 1 to 7) three times. It may take several days before the baby responds; he may expel gas on the first try. But his system will begin to function more and more smoothly, so that whenever he has an episode, a short massage will help break up and release trapped gas. Not every baby responds in the same way, and some, because of other factors, will not benefit as much as others. Many pediatricians now refer parents of gassy or colicky babies to infant massage instructors to address the problem without drugs.

Penny, mother of three-week-old Matthew, was nearly at the end of her rope with his colic; his pediatrician recommended she try massage, so she contacted me. When I first met Penny and Matthew, they were both so stressed by the colic that they had difficulty interacting with each other at all. "Matthew was very colicky until two weeks after I began massaging him, at which point the episodes began to subside," Penny said. "Within a few weeks, his colic disappeared completely. Now his disposition is very pleasant. He trusts me, and I have become much more relaxed." They were looking at each other, playing together, and Matthew was beginning to really enjoy being massaged. Even when Penny did the Colic Relief Routine, Matthew seemed to know how to cooperate and "work with it." With each round of strokes, he would wiggle and grunt and expel gas, and he responded well to the Touch Relaxation techniques.

Other aids may include warm baths, glycerin suppositories, and changes in diet. If you are nursing, eliminate irritants such as tomatoes, chocolate, caffeine, and gas-producing beans and vegetables. Sometimes a milk, soy, or wheat allergy can cause colic; try eliminating one or all of these, one at a time, from your or your baby's diet, and see if there is any change in her discomfort.

Seeing your little one in such distress isn't easy, and it can be terribly draining both physically and emotionally. "Being able to massage my baby and help him relax gave me peace of mind," says Mary, mother of eighteen-month-old Michael. "I started massaging him when he was two weeks old and having painful gassy

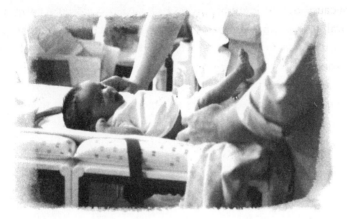

spells, and I saw results within a week. When he woke up crying in the middle of the night, I would massage him. After only a week, he would begin to relax as soon as I started stroking him. He would calm down and start releasing; often he fell asleep before I finished. I felt so good, being able to do something to help him, not to mention the extra hours of sleep it gave me! Even now, when he gets tense and out of sorts, I can talk to him and stroke him a little, and he relaxes. I wouldn't have known what to do for him otherwise. His infancy could have been just a disaster for all of us."

When my first baby was a newborn, he was very colicky. That was when I invented the Colic Relief Routine, adapting yoga techniques and advice from massage therapists to a baby's body. Within two weeks, his colic had resolved. But he remembered. When he was able to talk, he would request that I massage his tummy when he had gas pains, and he remembered to pull his knees up between strokes! This routine works for adults, too, and you may want to try it on yourself. Yoga practitioners use a similar pose, called *bhastrikasana* or Bellows Pose, upon waking in the morning, as it tones the gastrointestinal system and keeps the body regularly assimilating and eliminating as it should.

Because of the incredible stress of having a colicky baby, it is natural to feel somewhat negative and discouraged. But anyone who isn't feeling well does better when lovingly touched and cared for. Your baby is no exception. Massage can be a way to help your baby and thus boost your feelings of confidence and your self-esteem. This will not only make you a better parent, it will help your baby feel more secure, cry less, sleep more deeply, and bond with you completely. It's worth a try.

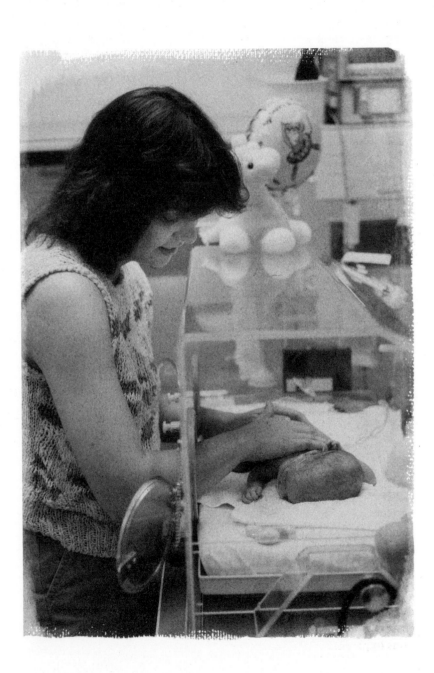

Chapter 11

Your
Premature Baby

Mother, let us imagine we are travelling,
and passing through a strange
and dangerous country.
 —Rabindranath Tagore

W E KNOW HOW important it is to hold our babies close, right from the start. We put a lot of planning into those first few hours and weeks, arranging to avoid the interruptions that would unnecessarily deprive our babies of those precious moments of bonding time.

When a baby arrives into the world long before she is expected, the best-laid plans are obliterated. The quiet, warm, joyous welcome hoped for is abruptly replaced by a kind of violence we never imagined. It is an unavoidable violence, one that keeps the baby alive but also engenders a tremendous range of feelings and reactions in parents.

Parents are thrust into cycles of grief: shock, denial (often manifesting as an obsession with the baby's medical condition rather than his recovery), guilt ("What did I do to cause this?"), anger (at baby, at spouse, at medical personnel, at fate), depression (often creating distance between the parent and the baby), bargaining ("I'll be the best parent ever if he just pulls through"), and fear. These feelings and many variations on them are natural and may recur in cycles for a long time after the baby's birth. Parents recover from the initial shock at different rates: most finally do accept the situation and try to find ways to help their baby through it and initiate the bonding process.

What about the premature baby? Thrust into cycles of her own—shock, pain, fear, withdrawal—she may be ignored as an emotional, feeling human being while the adults around her focus on lifesaving. This kind of treatment sometimes extends far beyond what is necessary, objectifying the baby and pushing an emotional wedge between her and her parents—between her and the world.

The preemie's first contact with human touch may bring pain: needles, probes, tubes, rough handling, bright lights—all sudden, after the warm protection of the womb. One of the first things parents can do to help and to begin bonding is to touch and hold their baby. This wonderful expression of caring contributes to both physical and psychological healing, not only for babies but for parents, too. Much of the anguish of those first days and weeks can be minimized if parents can feel some sense of control.

Many studies have proven that premature babies who are regularly stroked and who regularly hear their parents' voices during their nursery stay improve rapidly in growth and development. Judith Talaba, head nurse in a neonatal intensive care unit, has introduced massage and holding methods as a regular part of every baby's routine; many hospitals around the world do this now as a matter of course. "Massage gives parents a focus on the baby as an individual who needs her parents just as much as she needs the technology," Talaba says. "Parents in our nursery have become less concerned with oxygen concentrations, weight gain, and intake amounts, and more concerned about their infants being touched and massaged—a wonderful change of focus." Preemies in the intensive care unit have responded positively to massage, she adds, losing their hyperflexia (contraction of the body) and "withdrawing from touch" behaviors. Many have also had fewer apnea (cessation of breathing) spells.

Dr. Tiffany Field has done the most extensive studies of the effects of daily massage on premature babies. Her studies have shown that when these infants were massaged every day, a number of wonderful results followed: The babies spent more time in the active alert and awake states; cried less; had lower cortisol levels (indicating less depression); and went to sleep faster after massage than they did after rocking. Over a six-week period, the massaged babies gained weight, improved on emotionality, sociability, and soothability temperament tests, had decreased urinary stress hormones, and had increased levels of serotonin (one of the brain's natural pain relievers). The babies were able to leave the hospital earlier, saving thousands of dollars for parents, hospitals, and insurance companies.

MASSAGING YOUR PREMATURE BABY IN THE HOSPITAL

Preemies love the feeling of enclosure that a pair of warm, loving hands can give. But it is important to go very slowly, very tenderly. Before beginning a regular routine of massage, look around your baby's environment. What changes might be made to help your baby relax and feel more comfortable, less invaded? Sometimes a small change in light, sound, or handling can make a big difference.

A certain amount of light is necessary for the nurses to be able to observe the baby, but most nurseries will allow you to shade the baby's sensitive eyes. If your child is on a warming table, you can shield her head with an overturned box (such as a diaper box) with holes cut in all sides. In an incubator, a folded towel on top will do the trick. When the baby has stabilized, you can request that the incubator be shaded at night to help your baby regulate to cycles of day and night.

For a stark example of how our society objectifies infants, observe an adult intensive care unit and then a neonatal unit. The adult area is calm and quiet. But often the babies are subjected to loud conversation, ringing telephones, and rock music. Additional noise may include the high decibels of incubator monitors, the clatter of instruments and clipboards, and the slamming of incubator doors. You can ask nursery staff to lower the tone of conversation and music. You can fasten a sign on the incubator requesting gentle closing, and place a towel on top to dampen the clang of instruments.

Sounds that help your baby feel more comfortable can be introduced. Premature babies, like all babies, are soothed by their mother's voice and heartbeat sounds. When you are unable to be present, a heartbeat soother (available at many baby stores and through catalogs) may be introduced and, at intervals, a recording of your voice. First check it out with your baby; be sure the volume is low and not distressing. When you are there, talk and sing to her. Even if she doesn't seem to respond, she is listening. She remembers your voice, and it soothes her.

Your little one's first reactions to handling may be distressing. Go slowly: watch, listen, and learn from her and from sensitive hospital staff. A preemie's distress signals, which include apnea (cessation of breathing) and bradycardia (reduced heart rate), can instill so much fear that you may find yourself making excuses not to handle her.

In actuality and not surprisingly, studies show that mothers are the ones who are best able to reduce their preemies' distress. Breathe deeply, relax, and move through these moments with your baby. Assure her that she is okay, that you are here to love and care for her no matter what happens. Your baby needs to feel your strength and confidence.

Observe your infant's alertness cycles to decide when the best time may be for massage. Discover what kinds of stimulation she can handle. Some babies are extremely fragile and can cope with only one modality at a time—touching, talking, or eye contact, but not all three at once. Find out what kinds of drugs your baby has been given. Some (such as curare and pavulon) will make her unresponsive. Even then, your baby is aware of you, can feel and hear you, and needs your loving touch.

HOW TO BEGIN

You can begin your baby's massage routine with a simple daily dose of warm touch, the Resting Hands. This method is best while your baby is hospitalized; you can begin regular massage strokes when you bring him home from the hospital. Hold his tiny body in cupped hands, with a feeling of heaviness and deep relaxation in your hands. Practice your Controlled Belly Breathing. Feel relaxation and warmth in your hands. Respect your baby's communication, however subtle it may be. The nursery staff can help you learn his body language or cues, so you know when he needs a break from stimulation.

Conveying respect is an important part of infant massage. While he is forming initial feelings about himself and his body, whatever you reflect back to him will be taken seriously. This does not mean that, if the baby gives a signal that you interpret as negative, you must abruptly stop the massage. You want to help your child work through his fears, not reinforce them.

For example, babies who keep their arms tightly held to their

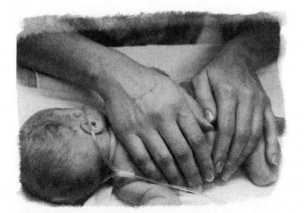

chests are indicating a need to protect this area of the body. Rather than pry the arms apart, hold them in their contraction with deep relaxation. Later, when you begin the massage strokes, stroke in the direction of the contraction. This tells the baby, "I support your need to protect yourself. I am on your side." Of course, you want to watch for signs that the baby has had enough and not go beyond what he can accept.

EYE CONTACT

A powerful connection is made when your baby first looks into your eyes. Eye contact is one of the important components in the dance of bonding, and one of the joys of massage. But preemies, because they are not yet ready to regulate themselves, need your help. Your baby may avoid eye contact altogether. You can gently offer encouragement by reducing harsh lights and positioning the baby so that you are accessible. Or your baby may become "locked in"—unable to release herself from looking and eventually becoming overstressed. If this happens, you can gently unlock her gaze after a moment or two by moving aside, passing a hand in front of her face, or shifting her position.

As your baby grows, her ability to communicate with you

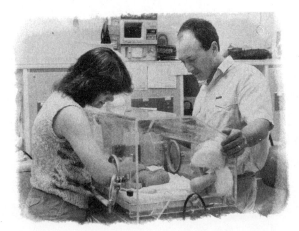

through eye contact will grow. Be patient, and don't force it. With slow and steady encouragement, you will soon treasure this important part of your bond.

TROUBLE SPOTS

Premature babies' bodies have been traumatized. Observe which areas of your baby's body may be especially programmed for pain. Often the feet, head, and chest are quite sensitive. At first, you may not be able to get to some of these areas because of the equipment. When you can reach them, begin like this:

1. Hold the baby's foot (head, chest, and so on) in your hands as if you were cupping a precious gem between your palms.

2. Deeply relax all over, taking several belly breaths. Let this relaxation move from your heart, through your arms and hands, to your baby.

3. Talk to the baby about relaxing his feet. Acknowledge that he has had a lot of pain in this area, and that he has been very courageous. You are here to help him release the pain and let pleasure in. Let him know that soon this painful time will be over, and he will be healthy and happy, ready to do what he wants to do in life. As you gently rock the area back and forth, use some key word or phrase such as "relax," or "let go."

4. When the baby responds with relaxation, praise his effort.

Repeat these steps every day, if possible, until you feel that the baby may be ready for more. Then you can begin gently massaging the area with oil, using the same relaxation and affirmation throughout.

STRESS CUES

Some researchers have found that babies in intensive care give cues to indicate they are stressed out that tend to be universal; these may not all apply to *your* baby, so use the nurses' knowledge and your own intuition to let you know what applies to your baby and when. These cues can include skin mottling, hiccups, gagging, apnea, bradycardia, and gestures of turning away or raising a hand up in front of her face as if she is warding off incoming stimuli.

These signs do not mean you should immediately stop Touch Relaxation or massage. Give the baby a break, then use the Resting Hands technique. If the baby continues to show signs of distress, let her sleep and try again later. Remember to breathe deeply and relax, and do not allow anyone to make you feel incompetent to care for your baby. Gradually, your baby's stimulation threshold will rise, and you will be able to touch and massage her more and more.

MASSAGING YOUR PREMATURE BABY AT HOME

You can really begin to work with your baby when he comes home from the hospital. Keep in mind that it is quite a change for him, and

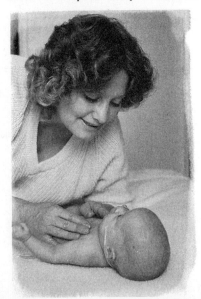

that he may regress a little. You may have to back up a bit with the massage, again focusing on relaxation and release.

In the warmth and security of your home environment, your baby will at last be able to release the tension and trauma of the hospital stay. This can be frightening and difficult for parents; suddenly the baby may be crying all the time. You may feel a little insecure without the hospital staff, as much as you may have previously resented their intrusions. At a time when you need reassurance, your baby's feedback seems to be "I don't like it here!"

Actually, the intense crying, if not caused by pain, is a healthy release. Often a baby will cry especially hard after a massage. This does not mean that he dislikes it or that you are doing it incorrectly. It is simply the only way available to him to release all his pent-up anguish. You can support your child by trying to relax and allow him to do what he needs to do, by being there to lovingly comfort him, and by trying to release your own fears. If you feel like crying with the baby (who wouldn't?), go right ahead.

Eventually you will progress from simple relaxation and holding to massage. Still, there are differences between massaging a premature baby and massaging a full-term infant. Begin by massaging the place on the baby's body that has been least invaded—usually the back. Miniaturize every stroke. Follow the strokes in Chapter 8, and simply modify them; for example, use two or three fingers instead of the whole hand. But do not be afraid to be firm. Your baby loves to feel the strength of your presence; a feathery touch can be overstimulating and irritating.

Be sure the space is very warm and that the baby is enclosed (use the Cradle Pose, or support the baby with firm pillows) and near you. You may want to warm the oil beforehand, but swishing it between your palms should be sufficient. Soon just the sound of the oil between your palms will cause your baby to open up like a little flower. He will learn to anticipate being massaged as a pleasurable experience, a time to feel the security of your loving hands. Once the tension is out of his body, his system will regulate. You will find marked improvement in his sleeping, feeding, digestion, and elimination, and you will notice a decrease in crying. Watch your baby bloom open to acceptance of life.

If possible, schedule yourself for an all-body massage by a competent, licensed therapist. You, too, have been through quite an ordeal. If you can release your own tensions and trauma, your baby will respond more positively to your touch.

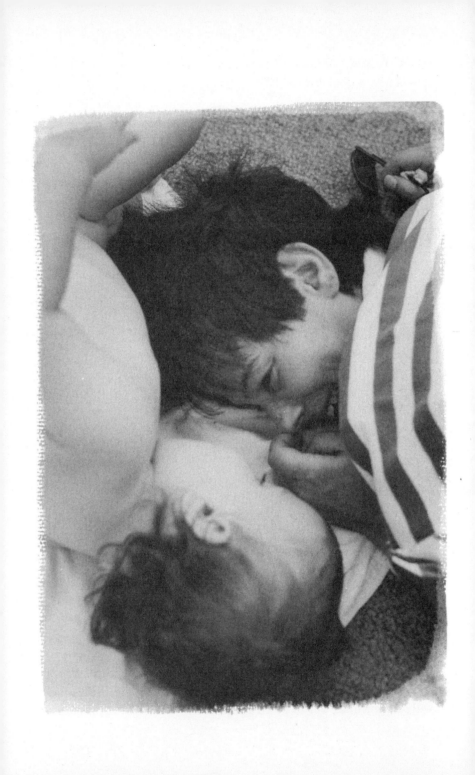

Chapter 12

Your Baby with Special Needs

The neighbor calls him a mongoloid;
The doctor says Down Syndrome.
I call him Kim.
　　　　　　—Mia Elmsater,
　　　　　　certified infant
　　　　　　massage instructor trainer

BONDING AND ATTACHMENT WITH SPECIAL BABIES

BONDING IS A MATTER OF reciprocal interaction. It depends upon a parent stimulating the infant with appropriate cues or signals, which trigger a response in the infant. The infant's cues or signals then trigger further involvement by the parent, including eye contact, smiling, speech sounds, and body movements. The baby with mental, visual, hearing, or developmental impairments or delays sometimes cannot respond in the ordinary manner to parental cues. Interactional synchrony thus may be inhibited, which can lead to the parent feeling out of touch with her baby. In addition, parents of babies with special needs are often overwhelmed by all of the information they need to absorb, by the therapies they are expected to carry out, and by the double bind of grieving and celebrating a new baby at the same time.

Parents' emotional reactions to the discovery of a special need in their newborn differ greatly. They can include confusion, denial, guilt, anger, wishful thinking, depression, intellectualization, and acceptance. These natural feelings can overlap and recur as parent and child adjust to their life together and to each new stage of the baby's development.

Infant massage can be a wonderful bonding tool for parents and babies with special needs. While physiological benefits do accrue, the focus and goal of infant massage is the interaction and connection of these two people. It is something you do *with* your baby rather than *to* your baby. It is not another therapy but an opportunity to share your love. A daily massage connects parent and baby in a way that no other type of interaction can match. Babies with special needs benefit from this intimacy even more than other babies. Because some avenues of communication may not be open to them, their parents need to know them well: the way the body feels when tense or relaxed, the look and feel of the abdomen when gassy or not, the difference between pain and tension. Often such parents need to be acutely aware of their infants' bodies because life-threatening infections can arise. A parent who is attuned to the look and feel of her baby's body at all times will more likely be able to detect toxicity in the early stages.

Elizabeth has cystic fibrosis, and her mother is glad she learned infant massage when Elizabeth was an infant. "At first we didn't massage our baby every day," Elizabeth's mother says, "but the more we did it and saw how wonderfully she responded, it grew on us. Elizabeth doesn't have her problem with being cold anymore. (If she does, we give her a massage.) She does not have so much abdominal pain, and her whole body is relaxed. Now when we massage Elizabeth, we concentrate not so much on cystic fibrosis as on Elizabeth as a beautiful little human being, a person. Infant massage has helped us have a relationship with her that has gone beyond our expectations. . . . It gives us great hope."

In this chapter, we will be discussing some particular challenges and how the massage may be altered for various types of conditions. Of course, this chapter cannot tell you how to best use massage with your baby in various challenging situations since there are just too many types of challenges, and within those categories many different babies with varying needs. What I can do, however, is give you some general information and hints to start with, so you then can approach your baby's physician, occupational therapist, or physical therapist with a basic knowledge of infant massage.

Before beginning a massage routine with your baby, check with the baby's doctor and physical therapist. They will help you design the massage and relaxation to suit your baby's needs. The International Association of Infant Massage offers continuing education programs for certified infant massage instructors (CIMIs) who work with babies who have medical challenges. I encourage you to seek out a CIMI with this extra knowledge to help you work with caregivers to massage your special baby.

Then trust yourself. You know your child better than anyone else. You are his or her specialist, and a companion in a way no one else ever can be.

DEVELOPMENTAL CHALLENGES

Developmental challenges such as cerebral palsy manifest in many different ways. The child's physical therapist will use procedures that either inhibit (relax) or facilitate (stimulate) muscle tone. Inhibition lessens muscle tone, while facilitation increases it. Inhibitory techniques may include slow stroking, gentle shaking, positioning, rocking, and neutral warmth. Facilitating techniques may include icing, brushing, positioning, pressure, and vibration. The massage strokes in this book can be modified to either inhibit or facilitate: To inhibit, use long, slow, sweeping strokes and Touch

Relaxation; to facilitate, use a more vigorous stroking and more playful interactions such as bouncy rhymes and songs.

The massage can be delivered in the same sequence as the massage in Chapter 8, with the following changes. Stroking the bottom of the foot often causes a reaction of extension and tightening of the leg. If this occurs, in Under Toes, Ball of Foot, and Thumb Press, change the stroke so that pressure is exerted on the outside rather than on the balls of the feet. The Thumbs to Sides stroke is particularly helpful in improving and stimulating diaphragmatic breathing. Infants with developmental challenges often show signs of resistance when the shoulders are stroked. For the chest, begin with Resting Hands, then try just one stroke, such as the Butterfly stroke across the chest, which includes the shoulder, and gradually increase as the child's stimulation threshold rises. For the face, the Smile strokes aid lip closure to promote good swallowing. These are particularly good for babies who drool and breathe through the mouth. The facial massage is an excellent prelude to oral stimulation and feeding therapy for the child who is sensitive around the mouth. When doing the Colic Relief Routine, do not hold the knees against the stomach for more than a count of five, so as not to inhibit respiration.

Babies who are tactile defensive—that is, hypersensitive and reactive to skin contact—benefit from firm pressure and stroking. Warm baths and brisk rubbing with a terrycloth towel before massage can increase acceptance of skin-to-skin massage.

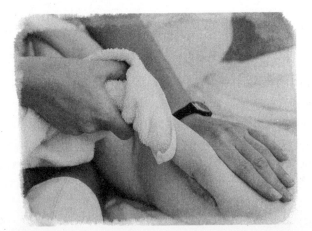

According to cerebral palsy experts, a slow, firm stroke down the center of the back can increase brain organization. Do not stroke up the back against hair growth.

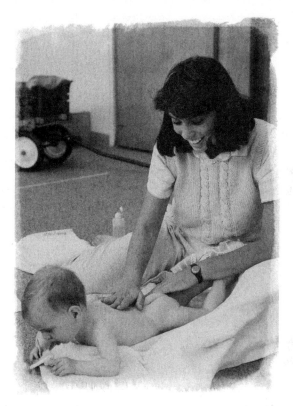

If your baby has a shunt or other type of bypass, her physical therapist will be able to tell you how much pressure is appropriate and how to work around these areas, even if at first the only thing you can do is use the Resting Hands technique on another part of the body such as the legs.

If your baby has had surgery, you can use massage, holding techniques, and Touch Relaxation with other parts of his body, with the support of his physician. Your loving touch and the security of it can be very important to your baby's recovery.

VISUAL CHALLENGES

Massage can be a particularly positive experience for babies with visual challenges because of their need for tactile stimulation as a means to define their world. Researchers have found remarkable results in both animal and human babies with visual challenges when tactile stimulation is used. One study reported that visual impairment did not produce a depression of emotional and learning behavior in animals if they received touch stimulation, whereas if this touch stimulation was withdrawn, they became either excessively passive or hyperaggressive. Other researchers have shown that babies in institutions who receive only twenty minutes of extra handling per day have significantly earlier development of visual attentiveness, indicating that the sensory system interlocks; the stimulation of touch does encourage visual exploration. Infants with visual challenges whose parents are particularly effective in establishing emotional bonds with them show a great deal of social interaction, perceptual attentiveness, and responsiveness in the first few months of life. These babies are able to reach toward sounds earlier than other babies with visual impairments.

Massage helps babies form an effective body image; this is important in establishing the object-constancy that allows the baby

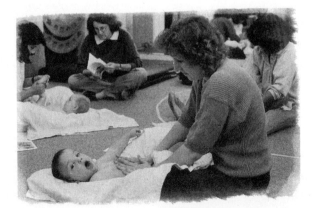

to let go of the parent and begin exploring the environment. In babies with visual challenges, motor development in the first few months is not different from that of babies with full sight, although there is often a lag in the onset of crawling and walking. Some researchers suggest that this may be due to the blind infant's resistance to lying prone, which may curtail the development of upper body strength, which is necessary for reaching and crawling. Massage in the prone position may gradually help the baby accept this position for play because massage becomes associated with trust and safety.

Your voice and touch simultaneously communicate love to your baby. Because you may not get the facial response you instinctively expect, you may find yourself withdrawing. Instead, find ways to develop an intimate rapport with your child through touch. Talk to your baby during the massage, explaining what you are doing and telling her what will happen next. Use her name often, and exaggerate auditory cues such as swishing the oil between your palms. During the first six months, do not use music or other sounds besides your voice. Later, music that imitates the rhythm of the strokes can be used as long as you interact with the music in a way that connects it to the massage, by singing or humming along, and stroking your baby to the music. Remain in close contact with the baby at all times during the massage. Keep your face close, and always keep one hand on his body. Always begin the massage with auditory cues and by gently holding and stroking the baby's legs and feet to initiate contact. Consider the light source during the massage. Light can be distracting to some babies with partial vision, while others need a stronger light source to feel comfortable.

AUDITORY CHALLENGES

Babies with hearing challenges have the same need for tactile comfort as other babies. Affectionate interaction is the most important element in any baby's life. Babies with auditory challenges need to be spoken to. During this early period, sound stimulates the growth of nerve connections between the baby's ear and brain. The sound stimulation in every baby's world creates an evolving network of nerve pathways. Many babies with hearing challenges are fitted with hearing aids to increase the amount of sound stimulation they receive. You can keep these on during the massage. The Infant Hearing Resource makes recommendations that might well be applied to all babies: "Tell the baby what you are thinking and feeling. He likes to hear about what makes you feel happy, sad, anxious, and excited. He can tell from the way you hold him and from your body language that you are experiencing different feelings. You might as well tell him what the names of those feelings are. Then, when he has different feelings, he will know what to call them."

Use normal speech with your baby during massage time, and make relaxed and loving eye contact with him as much as possible. Describe what you are doing. For example, "This is your foot, Jason. And here are your toes. One, two, three, four, five toes!" Converse with your baby and imitate his sounds. Experts agree that "parentese" or baby talk is a perfectly normal and acceptable form of communication with babies who have auditory challenges. Parents who choose to learn and teach sign language can begin during the massage, even before the baby can indicate comprehension of the signs.

Massage your baby for fun and enjoyment. There are many ways that a daily massage can enrich you, too. It will help you get to know your baby better, to feel more loving toward him, and to value his unique ways of communicating with the world.

MASSAGING BABIES WITH
SERIOUS MEDICAL CONDITIONS

The Touch Research Institute is continually replicating studies that prove that babies who have every imaginable problem—prematurity, HIV positive, cocaine exposure, depressed mothers, sexual and physical abuse, asthma, autism, diabetes, rheumatoid arthritis, developmental delays, eating disorders, dermatitis, cancer, burns, and post-traumatic stress disorders—all benefit from loving touch and massage. Massage in these cases has resulted in lower anxiety and stress hormones and improved scores on all clinical scoring methods.

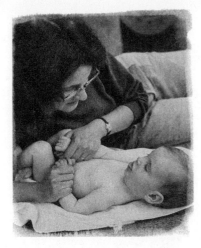

Generally, special precautions must be taken when massaging these babies, and the nursing staff can help you learn about these. Work with your baby's nurses, suggesting holding techniques such as the Resting Hands, carrying such as Kangaroo Care, and massage. If they don't know, contact your local certified infant massage instructor. If she or he does not have special training in this area, request that he or she find an instructor trainer who is familiar with this field and get the information you need. The references at the end of this book may help you, too. Remember, you are the parent or caregiver. You have the right to research and discover healthy ways to establish a strong bond of attachment with your baby.

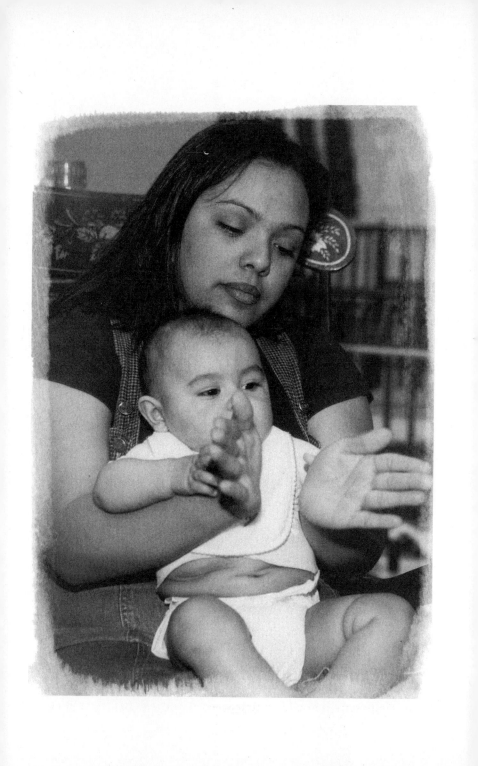

Chapter 13

Your Growing Child and Sibling Bonding Through Massage

The plants' bright blessing springs forth
From earth's gentle being,
And human children rise up
With grateful hearts to join
The spirits of the world.
—Rudolf Steiner

BIG KIDS NEED TOUCHING, TOO

ONE EVENING AFTER a family gathering at which a newborn cousin had made his first appearance, a friend's six-year-old daughter climbed into her mother's lap. "I wish I was a baby, Mommy," she said. "Then I'd get a lot of attention." That was a signal; time for a bedtime rubdown. Why? Not so much because she needed more attention, but because she needed to talk about the feelings her new cousin stirred in her.

It is important for children to talk about their feelings, but some-

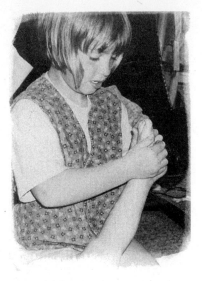

times it is difficult to get them to open up. Often, the more we question, the more unresponsive they become. My eight-year-old was to have surgery within a week, and though I knew he should talk about his fears, I hadn't yet been able to draw him out. The day after we had taken a tour of the children's ward and met the nurses at the hospital, he seemed tense. I asked him if he had any questions. "I dunno," he mumbled, shrugging his shoulders and slinking off to his room. Later that evening I offered him a foot massage. I gently massaged his calves, knees, and feet; within five minutes he relaxed and began to talk. He had several questions about the hospital and his surgery and was finally able to get the reassurance he needed—that I would be there with him, that he would not wake up during the surgery, and that he would be able to talk after his tonsillectomy. The operation went smoothly, and I remembered to use the soothing power of touch with him throughout the experience, before and after the surgery. A foot or hand massage now and then helped us both relax and let go of scary feelings.

Anthropologist Ashley Montagu, author of *Touching*, states that a child's close relationship with his parents is a source of basic self-esteem. "Persons who are callously unresponsive to human need, who have become so hardened that they are no longer in touch with the human condition, are not merely metaphorically so," he says, "but clearly physiologically so." A study reported in the *Journal of Humanistic Psychology* confirmed this idea, indicating that the higher the subject's self-esteem, the more he communicates through touch. Before the age of twelve, children are more tactile-kinesthetic—that is, they use feeling more than sight or hearing for information about the world. Therefore a warm touch can often trigger an outpouring of feeling or thoughts more than verbal communication. Saying "I love you" to your child is important, but more important is communicating your love through eye contact, through focused attention, and through your loving touch. In addition, for children, when praise is accompanied by touch, it is taken in eighty-five percent of the time, whereas praise given only with words is believed or absorbed only fifteen percent of the time.

Bonding between parents and children continues as the children age. Simply because a child has graduated from the in-arms stage doesn't mean she no longer needs your attention through healthy touching. She will no longer be nursing, she won't cuddle in the same way, her circle of support will widen, and she will be increasingly busy exploring the infinite possibilities of her world. But as she grows out of her mother's and father's arms, she will come to cherish those moments of closeness that reassure her that Mommy and Daddy are always there with a warm smile and a loving massage.

Though sometime in the first nine months is the ideal time to start the massage routine, it is never too late to begin. Usually a child between one and three years of age who has not been massaged from infancy will be much too busy to be still, but you may be able to start with a short, gentle backrub at bedtime. When the child becomes accustomed to being massaged, he will begin to

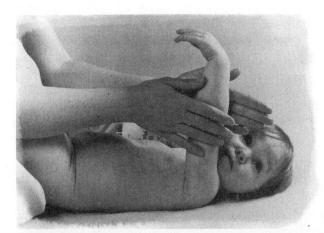

ask for it. Before you know it, he is massaging you! Ah, the universal law of action and reaction—what you do comes full circle back to you!

HOW TO BEGIN

Perhaps you've never considered massage as a means of opening communication between you and your child. How do you start without making it a "big deal"? The Soccer Player's Special (or ballerina's, whatever suits) is a good way to begin. Here's how:

1. Make sure the area is warm and comfortable with no distractions.

2. Wash your hands and remove jewelry.

3. Bedtime or after a bath is a good time, when your child is clean and ready to relax.

4. Always begin by asking permission, and respect your child's choices. Even when you move to another body part, you can say, "May I massage your tummy now?"

5. Use a natural oil, just enough to make your movements smooth without excessive oil.

6. Massage one leg at a time. Use the Milking and Rolling strokes (see Chapter 8). Use your thumbs to work circles around the knees, your fingertips to gently massage calf muscles, your thumbs to work all over the feet.

7. Build self-esteem by saying positive things about your child while massaging, such as "You have such beautiful hair" or "I noticed you shared your toys with your friend today. That was very nice of you. You are such a generous person."

AGES AND STAGES FOR MASSAGE

At different stages, your child will respond to being massaged differently. My best advice is to go with the flow, allowing her to lead you in the appropriate way. Here are some very common stages that children go through with massage, and what to do when your baby begins to respond differently. Of course, these ages are not rigid; each child will have his own rhythm and cycles of growth.

The Active Crawler

Active crawling is a challenging time for most parents, who are accustomed to massaging their infant as a soothing, quiet, communicative, and even meditative experience. When the baby starts crawling, massage becomes more playful and fun. Just about anything is preferable to lying on her back! You can use rhymes and games, give her a toy to play with or a hard biscuit to suck on. Instead of adhering rigidly to the sequence of stroking, just massage the part that appears in front of you. Babies will roll around, crawl, climb in your lap, sit up, and do all manner of movements. Be creative with your massage. My son and I made a game; he would start to crawl away, and I would say, "Oh, no you don't! I'm gonna get you now!" and laugh, pulling him back toward my lap. He would laugh and want to do this over and over again. In the meantime, I massaged his back, his buttocks, his legs, and his feet.

The Toddler

From age one to three, your child will be developing her autonomy, and a big part of autonomy is exercising her freedom to say "no." She may often reject massage altogether during this period. If this is her response when you offer a massage, respect her choice. Sometimes she may ask for a massage in a coded way, such as "I have a tummy ache." Then you can offer a tummy massage. You can do the strokes in a playful way. Clara Ute Zacher Laves, an IAIM instructor-trainer, suggests doing fun things like planting a garden on the child's back, or making a pizza on her tummy. Use your imagination, and your child will enjoy this opportunity for creative play. The Milking strokes should be done in two parts: first the thigh (or upper arm) and then the calf (or forearm). The Squeeze and Twist and Rolling strokes should start just below the knee or elbow rather than the hip or shoulder to prevent "twisting" the joint.

The Preschool Child

At about age three, your child will settle down and enjoy being massaged again in a more quiet way. Now that he has established his independence, he will like the feeling of being a "baby" again, receiving all of his parent's attention. You can massage after a bath or at bedtime. Adapt the strokes to the child's growing limbs, leaving out strokes that don't fit or seem appropriate. Respect the modesty your child may have developed by now, and allow him to keep his T-shirt and underwear on. Tell a story as you massage legs, feet, tummy, and back, or ask your child what body part you are massaging, helping him learn the names of different parts, such as forearm, thigh, calf, and so on. From now on, you can leave out the Gentle Movements, as your child is getting plenty of stretching and exercise in his day-to-day life.

The School-Age Child

Again, you will adapt the strokes to your child's growing limbs, kneading the thigh and calf muscles as she lies flat rather than using the Milking or Squeezing strokes. Offer open-ended questions or statements that will encourage her to talk, such as "It seemed like you were a little sad when you came home today." Music, storytelling, and talking can enhance the massage experience and allow time for your child to feel special and open up to you. You might add scent to your massage oil, allowing her to choose the scent. Most school-age children will enjoy the massage more if they are lying on their stomach rather than face-up.

The Adolescent

With adolescents, it is often hard to give a massage, as self-consciousness is high during this period. You can offer a foot or back massage as you talk to your child about his day. If he is open, you can then offer, "Would you like me to rub your calves?" During this period, stay away from body parts associated with sexuality, as your child will be uncomfortable with this and it is appropriate to keep boundaries intact as he grows into adulthood. Again, your adolescent will enjoy the massage more if he is lying on his stomach as opposed to face-up. Offer pillows under the stomach or other areas for comfort.

When your daughter begins menstruation, if she has cramps, you can massage her belly or lower back to ease her discomfort. Using the "heel" of your palm, push up the lower back at the tailbone to relieve cramps and pressure. Acupressure points at the Achilles tendon, just under either side of the ankle bone, can be massaged, which often relieves cramping. You can have her sit up on the floor between your knees, and knead tension from her neck and shoulders as you talk about whatever is on her mind. With her face turned away from you, it is easier for her to talk about her feelings and worries.

RHYMES AND GAMES FOR THE OLDER BABY

Massaging an older baby requires a different approach from massaging an infant. To keep the child interested and involved, you may want to vary the massage each time, adding stories, songs, and animation. For example, one of the tummy strokes most enjoyed by toddlers is I Love You (see page 89). They enjoy chiming in with you as you stretch the words out, cooing in a singsong voice. When you massage the feet, you can play "This little piggy went to market." Little games, songs, and stories that you invent as you massage your little one will involve him, entertain his active mind, and promote the kind of communication that stimulates and utilizes all of his developing senses.

Feet and Toes

This little piggy went to market
This little piggy stayed home
This little piggy had roast beef [*tofu? pomegranates?*]
This little piggy had none
This little piggy went, wee wee wee wee all the way home.

One is a lady that sits in the sun;
Two is a baby and three is a nun;
Four is a lily with innocent breast;
Five is a birdie asleep in his nest.

This little piggy got into the barn,
This one ate all the corn.
This one said he wasn't well,
This one said he'd go and tell,
And this one said—squeak, squeak, squeak!
I can't get over the barn door sill!

See saw, Marjorie Daw,
The hen flew over the barn.
She counted her baby chicks one by one,
    [*count each toe except the baby toe*]
But she couldn't find the little brown [*white*] one.
Here it is, here it is, here it is!

    [*start with the little toe*]
This little cow eats grass,
This little cow eats hay,
This little cow looks over the hedge,
This little cow runs away,
And this *big* cow does nothing at all
But lie in the fields all day!
We'll chase her, and chase her,
And *chase* her!

[This rhyme goes well with the foot strokes using the thumbs that press all over the foot; see pages 77–80.]

Pitty patty polt,
Shoe the wild colt.
Here's a nail,
There's a nail,
Pitty patty polt!

Tummy

[Use this rhyme with the Sun Moon stroke; see page 88.]

Round and round the garden
Went the teddy bear,
One step, two step, tickley under there!
[walk fingers up to armpit]

Fingers

Five little fishes swimming in a pool
[open hand]
First one said, "The pool is cool."
Second one said, "The pool is deep."
Third one said, "I want to sleep."
Fourth one said, "Let's dive and dip."
Fifth one said, "I spy a ship."
They all jumped up and went ker-splash
[stroke top of hand]
Away the five little fishes dash.
[gently wiggle hand to relax]

[begin with thumb]
This is the father, short and stout.
This is the mother, with children all about.
This is the brother, tall you see.
This is the sister with dolly on her knee.
This is the baby, sure to grow.
And here is the family, all in a row.

Here is a tree with leaves so green,
Here are the apples that hang between
    [hold baby's thumb and small finger and dangle
        three middle fingers]
When the wind blows the apples fall
    [hold baby's wrist and gently wiggle]
And here is a basket to gather them all.
    [cup baby's hand in yours]

Five little kittens
All black and white
    [cup baby's fist in your hands]
Sleeping soundly
All through the night
Meow, meow, meow, meow, meow
    [raise each finger]
It's time to get up now!

Within a little apple
So cozy and so small
There are five little chambers
    [cup baby's fist in yours]
Around a little hall.

In every room are sleeping
Two seeds of golden brown
They're lying there and dreaming
    [open each finger and peek in]
In beds of eiderdown.

They're dreaming there of sunshine
And how it's going to be
    [stroke top of hand]
When they shall hang as apples
Upon the Christmas tree.
    [hold baby's wrist and gently wiggle]

Face

Knock knock
    [Open Book stroke on forehead; see page 92.]
Peek in
    [gently open eyes with thumbs]
Open the latch
    *[with thumbs, push up on the bridge of nose and down
        diagonally across cheeks]*
And walk right in.
    [Smile strokes]
Hello, Mr. Chinny-chin-chin!
    [gently wiggle chin]

Two little eyes to look around
Two little ears to hear each sound
One little nose to smell what's sweet
One little mouth that likes to eat.

Peek-a-boo, I see you
Hiding behind the chair
Peek-a-boo, I see you
Hiding there.

GAMES TO PLAY WITH GENTLE MOVEMENTS

Arms

Up so high
    [stretch arms up]
Down so low
    [bring arms down]
Give a little shake
    [wiggle hands at wrists]
And hold them so.
    [put palms together]

This is my right arm, hold it flat.

[hold right arm out to the side, flat on surface]

This is my left arm, just like that.

[repeat with left arm]

Right arm

[bring right arm across chest]

Left arm

[bring left arm across chest to hug self]

Hug myself!

Left arm

[open out left arm again]

Right arm

[repeat with right arm]

Catch a little elf!

[bring palms together quickly, then ask, "Did you catch him?" and peek in cupped hands]

Pat-a-cake, pat-a-cake

[pat baby's hands together]

Baker man,

Bake me a cake as fast as you can.

[hold arms up, then down]

Roll it

[roll hands around each other]

And pat it

[pat palms together]

And mark it with a B

[make a B with baby's hand]

And put it in the oven

[hold arms up, then down]

For baby and me.

[point to baby and self]

Legs

One leg, two legs

[*cross legs over tummy, right leg on top*]

Hot cross buns

[*cross legs over tummy, left leg on top*]

Right leg, left leg

[*pull legs gently toward you, flat on surface*]

Isn't that fun?

[*gently wiggle legs to release tension*]

Up

[*knees into tummy*]

Down

[*gently pull legs out straight*]

Up

[*knees into tummy*]

Down

[*gently pull legs out straight*]

And shake them all around

[*gently wiggle legs to release tension*]

HELPING AN OLDER CHILD ADJUST TO A NEW BABY

A new baby is a fascinating, fearful creature to her older brother or sister. Hovered over and protected by adults, she seems an unapproachable, somehow dangerous little thing. Much has been written on the importance of letting your older child know that he is still loved and cherished in his own right when a new baby comes into the family. The next step is to help the older child and the baby begin a relationship of their own. It usually takes quite a bit longer for a child to fully bond with a new sibling. His first task is to understand that the baby is "here," that mother is all right, that he is still loved as much as before, and that life goes on.

As you massage your baby every day, your older child will occasionally observe. He may remember being massaged (in fact, he still may enjoy being massaged) and identify with the baby. They share an experience and have something in common.

If you give your child the opportunity to massage the baby occasionally (only if he wants to, of course), he will benefit by it in many ways, as will the baby. The older child will bond with the baby in the same ways that you do—with eye contact, touch, movement, and sound. He will learn that the baby is not necessarily so dangerous and fragile but a person like himself. His confidence will bloom as he comes to realize his own competence as a caregiver and protector. The baby will respond to him, overcoming her initial fear of his sometimes clumsy or rough handling, or startling behavior. She will begin to relate to him as a loving peer and ally.

It is best to delay suggesting that an older child massage the new baby until the baby has passed that stage of fragility when she is easily startled. Usually three or four months of age is about the right time, though a little earlier may be appropriate for an older child who is over four. Don't worry about the techniques or whether your child uses oil. You can show him a couple of simple things (like the Open Book stroke on the chest or the I Love You stroke on the tummy), and then let him do it as he pleases. He will at first be hesitant and

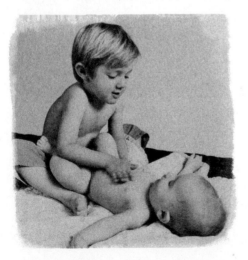

may need your encouragement to touch the baby. He might stroke her only a couple of times. But even the tiniest amount of contact will be very beneficial. Be sure to express your pleasure and pride to your child. Let him know that he did a good job and that his massaging is valuable to the baby.

HEALTHY TOUCH

Parents are concerned about the touching their children receive, and about helping them protect themselves from unhealthy individuals who may take advantage of them. Unfortunately, because of the fear engendered by newspaper stories of molested children, many parents are giving their children frightening, negative messages about touch.

It is important that our children know the difference between healthy and unhealthy touching. Infant massage is a great way to positively teach a child the difference. A child who has been massaged from infancy has several advantages over the child who is simply educated or warned about unhealthy or unwanted touch. The massaged child knows what healthy, loving touch feels like. Because of the emotional bonds it produces between parent and child, he feels close to his parents and tends to talk about his feelings more often. Thus, he would be much more likely to report to his parents if he were concerned about the way someone talked to him or tried to touch him. In addition, massage time becomes "talking time," a time when parent and child can discuss things that are important to both of them. It is a perfect opportunity to talk about touching with your older child, and to help him learn how to protect himself. You can tell him, "Always tell me or Daddy or your teacher if somebody tries to touch you in a way that you don't like. I promise, no matter what, you will be safe." The type of interaction afforded by regular massage and Touch Relaxation helps your child develop a positive self-image and a sense of ownership of his body. He also develops a keen awareness of feelings and body language. The respect we show in asking permission to massage and to move to different parts of the body teaches him that people should ask his permission for intimate touch.

In general, massaged children grow up feeling confident and comfortable in their bodies, and they openly communicate with their parents. It is a tradition with long-term benefits, and it is definitely worth the effort!

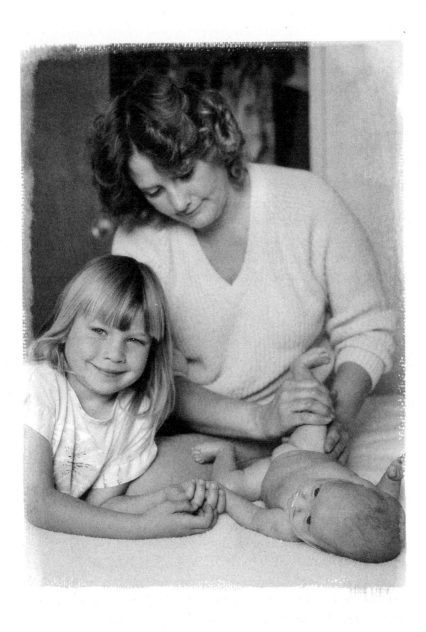

Chapter 14

Your Adopted or Foster Children

Not flesh of my flesh
Nor bone of my bone
But still miraculously my own.
Never forget for a single minute
You didn't grow under my heart,
But in it.

—Anonymous

ATTACHMENT

ADOPTIVE AND FOSTER PARENTS are some of the most loving parents in the world. They choose their children, often children with medical problems and/or impairments, or children from races and cultures other than their own. These parents have a great deal of love to give. Yet it is common for their babies and children to resist affection.

Some past bonding theories have suggested that true bonding may not be possible between parents and children who are adopted or fostered. But ample evidence now proves that adoptive and foster parents can bond and form the same kinds of attachments that biological parents and their children form. Researchers David Brodinsky, Leslie Singer, Mary Stein, and Douglas Ramsey, among others, have found no difference in the development of parents' attachment to adopted and biological babies of the same age. If adoptive or foster parents provide a familial atmosphere—a warm, affectionate, and consistent response to a baby's needs—trust is learned and an attachment develops.

Lois Melina, an expert on adoption issues, cautions adoptive parents not to be too eager and overwhelm their new baby with affection. Often babies who come from a foster home or an orphanage are resistant to touch and affection, as well as easily overwhelmed by it. In addition, they must grieve the loss of their previous caregivers and homes and be allowed to gradually become part of their new family and environment. Gail Steinberg, of the on-line group Pact, An Adoption Alliance, and the author of *Bonding and Attachment: How Does Adoption Affect a Newborn?*, says, "The best signals for knowing you're on track will come from the baby. Gather strength from simple pleasures: smiles and developmental milestones are proud signs of growth. Baby may take more or less time to attach than you do.

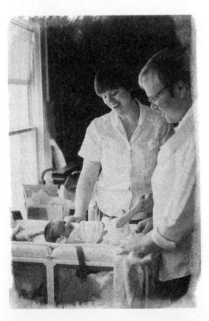

Your partner may take more or less time. It may take days, weeks, months, or a year. Don't feel like a failure if attachment takes longer than you imagined. Most important is building a family together, no matter how long it takes."

Entire articles have been written about what's been called Post-Adoption Depression Syndrome. Often adoptive parents go through months and even years of what author June Bond calls "infertility hell," then go through an often prolonged adoption process. After the wonderful first days or weeks of having your new baby at home, it is not uncommon for one or both parents to experience feelings of anxiety, inadequacy, confusion, and a kind of letdown blues. Often when we reach a long-held goal, we experience anticlimax—the natural loss of the high arousal felt on the way to reaching a goal. You may also contend with feelings of guilt for the birth mother's grief and loss, stress from the expense,

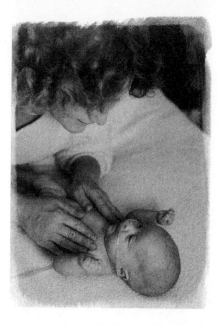

and perhaps dismay at discovering previously unknown or undisclosed health problems and background information about your child. Often adopted babies have attachment disorders, difficult adjustment periods, and overwhelming needs. Just like a biological parent, you may go through emotional ups and downs, lack of sleep, increased responsibilities, and stress levels. Joining an adoptive parents' support group helps some parents feel validated; sharing your feelings with others can help you realize other people have similar concerns. People further down the road can help you see that these feelings change, recognize developmental milestones, and avoid the difficulties that many first-time parents experience.

The new baby will experience both the normal stresses and the added stress of adjusting to a new environment, new caregivers, new sights, sounds, smells, tastes, and rhythms. Sometimes a newly adopted baby regresses for a time, withdraws from touch, and eventually cries deeply and uncontrollably. Read Chapter 9 again and use all your listening skills to help your baby grieve and cry in the safety of your love. Often babies won't begin to fuss and cry until they feel safe to do so—you can consider it a positive milestone when your baby or child begins to express his grief, anger, or even rage around you. Remember this as your baby grows older, for these feelings can surface again and again, and the best thing you can do is listen, allow venting to occur, and let your child know he is loved without condition.

MAKING TRANSITIONS

Try to find out as much as you can about the baby's previous environment and caregiving routine, who took care of her, what her birth was like, what formulas or foods she was given, and what colors, sounds, and smells she is accustomed to. Try to replicate some of these to allow her the comfort of the old while adapting to the new. For example, adoption expert Anna Marie Merrill suggests the following, which I hope will spark ideas about how to create a transitional environment for your baby:

❖ If a foster mother or previous caregiver used a certain perfume or scent, put a dab on a hanky for the baby's crib or rest place.

❖ If the baby is accustomed to a propped bottle, prop her bottle, but hold her while she is being fed.

❖ Begin eye contact by playing peek-a-boo and other eye contact games that give the baby a chance to make brief eye contact, feel its safety, and gradually move to more extended interaction.

❖ If the baby is used to being swaddled, use swaddling at home to help him bring his energies to center after a period of grief-release crying.

❖ For older babies, put food (such as Cheerios) into her mouth with your fingers instead of having her pick them up. This allows a little skin-to-skin contact, building trust.

❖ If the baby seems to withdraw from touch, try the Resting Hands technique for a while before trying massage. When you do begin the massage, emphasize the permission period and carefully watch your baby's cues. Be sure you are deeply relaxed yourself, and focused softly on him. If even Resting Hands is too much, step back further, perhaps leaving the clothing on and holding his legs or feet for a very short period. Gradually work up from there as your baby's cues indicate he is ready for more.

❖ Learn about the music, songs, or sounds the baby may have been accustomed to hearing and feeling in her previous environment, and use them during short periods throughout the day.

❖ Many countries water down formula or add a lot of sugar to it. Though you may not agree with these practices, you can begin using the same formula, gradually increasing the substance and decreasing the sugar or water content. Be aware of lactose intolerance; many babies from countries outside developed countries or who have been breastfed may react poorly to the rich cow's milk we drink in the West.

❖ Instead of those crisp, new baby clothes you'd love to dress your new child in, find some soft, well-worn used clothing. Try to find out about and obtain the same laundry soap that was used in the baby's previous environment. The clothing will then smell familiar to him. Cut labels from the back of the clothing, which may feel scratchy and irritating.

❖ If your baby has come from an orphanage where all the walls were painted bright, sky blue, you might consider painting her room the same color for a while.

These types of transitional changes can help the baby feel more open to his new surroundings and less fearful, with familiar sights and sounds to soothe him. Anna Marie agrees that it is important to allow adopted and foster babies time to grieve. Do not hush every fuss or cry, but rather talk to the baby, allowing him to cry out his frustrations, fears, anger, grief, pain, and loneliness. If children are not allowed to do this in infancy (and sometimes even when they are), they will often act out violently when they are older, when they know it is "safe enough to misbehave." They will test you to see if you still love them when they are not on their best behavior.

Your new baby may be able to handle only one or two sources of stimulation at a time, so don't overload her by singing, massaging, having a television on in the background, and so on. Present one interaction at a time, such as eye contact or singing or massage, but do not combine them until she is ready.

Gail Steinberg suggests continuing to show affection to your new baby, even though he may arch, stiffen, and seem to reject it. But don't force him. If eye contact is threatening, try small doses from a distance, and allow your baby to watch you when you change his clothing, feed, and bathe him without necessarily looking back. Allow him to gradually develop comfort with closeness.

One story, told to me by Anna Marie Merrill, demonstrates beautifully how one creative mother used this gradual process to achieve closeness with her adopted older son. She had a scarf and made a game wherein she would hold one end of the scarf, the boy the other. She would pull the scarf toward her just a tiny bit, and then wait until he did so, too. It took a long time, but eventually their hands met, and the safety of attachment had been achieved. Another mother used story time as a way to introduce her child to touch in a noninvasive and nonthreatening way. Each day at a cer-

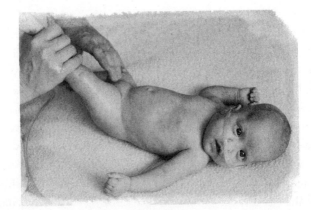

tain time she read the child a story as they sat in a rocking chair. Because the focus was on the story, the child could accept the physical contact.

Sometimes an adoptive or foster baby becomes attached to one parent but rejects the other. In this case, it is important for the rejected parent to find very gentle, slow methods to create the safety necessary for attachment. Merrill suggests that "nurturing dependence" is the beginning of creating attachment. So good things for the rejected parent to do would be to change, feed, or bathe the baby, if the baby can accept it. If not, give the baby some time and try again. Trust builds over time, and your mere consistent, accepting presence will foster the beginning of attachment cues to which you can respond.

MASSAGING THE ADOPTED OR FOSTERED BABY

Massaging an adopted or fostered baby is needed but can also be very difficult. Adoption expert Renée Henning says, "I do not want to overstate the difference between a baby from foster care or an orphanage and the average baby. There may be no difference in numerous cases. However, many babies from foster homes or orphanages do need good touching more than the average baby. Yet some of these babies may be initially less receptive to massage or less able to enjoy an extended massage than the average baby."

My suggestion is that you begin very slowly, using Resting Hands, with the baby fully clothed, and gradually move toward the entire massage presented in this book. Remember that your baby needs to grieve, and your best response is to validate her feelings and continue to offer loving touch, backing up when you need to, then moving forward again as trust and attachment grow. Nancy Verrier, in "Healing the Primal Wound," says: "Children are creatures of sensation and intuition, and they know whether or not there is permission for them to experience and/or express their feelings." She stresses the importance of allowing your new baby to cry and feel understood. Often massage can help the baby begin to release these pent-up feelings of grief and fear.

Adoption expert Marlou Russell emphasizes the importance of finding this release. "Since loss is such a major part of adoption, grieving is a necessary and important process," she says. "Adoption can create a situation in which grieving is delayed or denied. Because adoption has been seen as such a positive solution, it may be difficult to feel that it is okay to grieve." This grief, when allowed—even encouraged—in infancy can help diminish later behavioral problems stemming from unresolved emotional pain. According to Leah LaGoy, another of Pact's on-line authors on adoption issues, the teenage years can restimulate the grief suppressed in babyhood because adolescence is a time of major transition and identity crisis. Teenagers often become angry at their adoptive parents; at least some of this is repressed rage at the birth parents, whom they may unconsciously or consciously feel abandoned them.

If your adopted or foster baby responds negatively to your affectionate overtures, she may have some attachment or bonding disorder that can and should be addressed as soon as possible. The baby may not have received the response she needed in her previous environment, and she may have given up trying to get her needs met. When affection and responsiveness are finally offered, she may very likely react with stiffening, refusal to be consoled, and irritability. Don't take these behaviors personally. Validate the baby's feelings, and find ways to continue offering her loving touch and affection until she feels safe enough to relax into your love and accept your nurturing, including massage. All experts on attachment disorders stress the importance of addressing these issues as early in the baby's life as possible to prevent problems from surfacing later, be they social problems at school or pathological, sociopathic behavior. The older a child becomes, the more difficult it is to "rewire" the brain so as to be able to create and sustain healthy, interdependent, and loving relationships.

When teaching infant massage to foster parents, I am often

asked, "Should I really massage this baby and help him resolve his grief, when he may be sent back into an abusive or neglectful situation?" My response is a resounding "yes!" Releasing his grief and fear, and accepting and experiencing healthy affection and attachment, can help the baby be more resilient, healthier, and more independent. If he is sent back to abusive caregivers, his behavior with them may be different, causing a different response from them. For example, he may be more relaxed, smile more, be more "cuddly," and initiate eye contact more often. These behaviors can influence the caregivers to feel more loving and responsive toward him, thus changing their relationship and building more trust. If the caregivers can be taught good parenting skills and healthy, correct infant massage, so much the better.

As Terry Levy and Michael Orlans conclude, "The studies on attachment patterns, development and psychosocial functioning consistently show that children classified as securely attached in infancy do better in every important area of life as they develop." They show that these children solve problems more competently, are more resilient, make better friends, have higher self-esteem, are more independent, and receive more positive feedback from their environment.

Massaging your baby, whether you are an adoptive or a foster parent, can be one of the best things you can do for both yourself and your child, to create loving, relaxed, open, healthy bonds that will stay with your baby for his or her entire life. What an incredible gift you can give: a legacy that can change the interactions of generations to come.

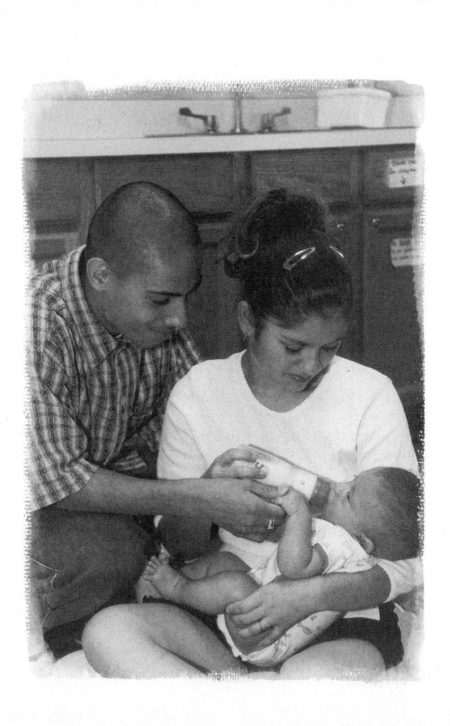

Chapter 15

A Note to Teen Parents

I F YOU HAVE DECIDED to keep and raise your baby, you have made a very difficult choice, not only for yourself but for many of your loved ones, including your baby. If you have made that choice, I respect it, and I hope you have adults in your life who respect your choices and will support and help you. It is of utmost importance to both your future and that of your baby that you gather as much loving support and help from adults as you can. Don't let someone

---

To Older Parents:
This small chapter is difficult for me, but I feel it is important to acknowledge teen parents and encourage them in the good things they want to do for their babies. I am in no way condoning or encouraging teen pregnancy; anyone who has had children and raised them to adulthood knows that it would be foolish to do so. But neither am I blind to the reality that many teens become pregnant and decide for their own reasons to keep their babies. Rather than punishing them, I believe education, support, and assistance in being the best parents they can be is the best choice we as adults can make.

discourage you—just move on and keep searching out those people who can make up your little "village," for in this case it truly does take a village to raise a child. You will find yourself trying to navigate some pretty complicated waters. The decisions you will have to make will seem endless at times. Your body is constantly changing, and discomforts you never expected can make you irritable. Everyone has an opinion or advice to offer, some more destructive than constructive.

Whatever people say, you have made a choice, consciously or not, to become an adult before your biological programming or the culture may be ready for it. Stresses of education, family, relationships, physical discomforts, body image concerns, self-esteem, friendships, and medical issues can seem to bear down on you all at once. I won't try, here, to cover all of the issues you are dealing with. What I want to do is stress that your love for your baby has to become your number-one priority, and whatever supports that should be kept close and healthy. Whatever doesn't—for the time being—put on the back burner or remove from your life.

I encourage you to get good prenatal care, listen to your doctors, and read as much as you can about every aspect of this new phase of your life. Your baby's life and health—and yours—may depend on it. Take control of your life and with calm determination create a warm, safe, and loving environment into which you bring your baby and nourish your own spirit. If your mother isn't available, seek out the best mother you can think of and have the courage to ask her to help you be a good parent, even if it's only with occasional hugs, a listening heart, and answers to baby-care questions on the phone.

Massage is a great way to learn who your baby is and to begin the biological process that will create a loving and unbreakable bond between you. Even if you can't do it every day, try to find some way to work it in as a weekly or every-other-day ritual after your baby is born. Take an infant massage class from a certified instructor if you can find one.

Remember the elements of the bonding process, and try to get them all covered every day:

- ❖ Have skin-to-skin contact with your baby.
- ❖ Make warm and loving eye contact.
- ❖ Talk and play with your baby.
- ❖ Look at your baby's face when nursing or feeding him.
- ❖ Carry the baby on your chest for a little while each day.
- ❖ Avoid strong perfumes or scents the first three months.

Other important things to remember in those sleep-deprived months of early parenting:

- ❖ Never leave the baby alone or with people who you know are unreliable or uneducated in baby care.

- ❖ Never punish a baby either verbally or physically, and never use profanity in talking about or to your baby. If you feel stressed out and need some time to yourself, try to find someone to watch her for a little while. Fifteen minutes for a walk or deep breathing, or even dancing to your favorite music, can help get you in a better mood.

- ❖ Remember that crying is just a baby's way of talking, and they sometimes have a lot to talk about. Never isolate the baby or punish her for crying.

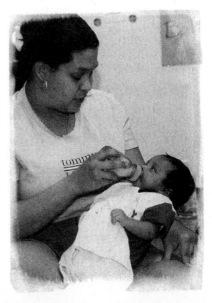

Other things you can do are covered in this book, particularly the chapters about crying and fussing, colic, and attachment. What

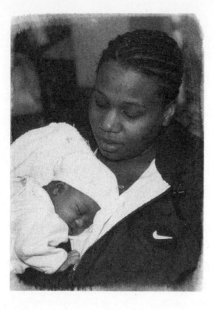

you do the first year or two will lay a foundation for an entire lifetime. For teens, a year or two seems like a long time, and I won't kid you—sometimes it's really hard and demands a lot more sacrifice than you thought. But hang in there. This is happening in your life for a reason, and later on you will be so glad and proud of yourself for being a good parent when it really counted. Beginning this way, you will get hooked on the wonderful "high" of being a good parent and find strengths you never knew you had. Your child will look to you to know how to be a good person, and being your child's role model will become an education in itself as you seek out the knowledge you need and continually improve yourself so your child will look to you with pride.

All my best wishes go with you on this incredible journey of creating a family.

FOR TEEN FATHERS

As you already know, it takes more than making a baby to father a child. If you and your partner are having a baby, I encourage you to stay as close as possible to your baby. Even if you and your partner are not together anymore [if she has decided not to put the baby up for adoption], you can cooperate in coparenting. Try to make the environment as stress-free as possible for the baby's mother, setting your ego aside for the sake of your child. Gather strength from any adult male role model you can find, be he your own father, a pastor, a counselor or coach at school, or a counselor from your local social services agency. [Read the books and resources suggested in "References and Recommendations," and take an active part in the entire process as much as you are able.] You will be required to sacrifice a lot of what you may want for yourself in order to provide financial support for your family. But don't make the mistake of thinking that financial support can take the place of loving bonds.

If your partner is punitive or uncooperative, do whatever it takes, including cooperating in counseling sessions together, to cool down the emotional temperature and humble yourself so that you will have a chance to be a good father to your baby. Take whatever classes or workshops may be offered to you. Show your partner you are making your best effort to support your child both financially and emotionally. This can be a very difficult and stressful time for all of you. But I implore you, if at all possible, to be an active, every-day part of your baby's life. It will be one of the most important things you do in your life, one that you will look back upon with no regrets when you are older. A solid, loving relationship with your child will enable both you and your child to succeed and be happy in the future. If you are fathering a child, there is no doubt about it—ready or not, it's time to grow up. And I assure you, the joy you get from your child's love will be worth every effort you make to be a good, solid, loving, responsible father and role model.

If your partner decides to put the baby up for adoption, many states now have "open adoptions," and you can find out how best to be involved as the baby's biological father. We are all realizing that the physical, emotional, mental, and spiritual well-being of our babies must come first and foremost, and we must be willing to sacrifice at the proper time, to step forward at the proper time, and never to abandon our children, regardless of the final outcome. It is a lot to ask, but you can do it if you make up your mind that it is what you want and need, both for yourself and for your baby.

REFERENCES AND RECOMMENDATIONS

You will notice many of these studies are very old. That is because often they were the first groundbreaking studies that have since been proven over and over again. I feel the first studies are the most important, and they are the ones from which I drew my conclusions, so I do not list here every study that has been done on the subject since then. In addition, in a book such as this one, footnotes are distracting. Therefore, the studies I refer to in the text are listed by chapter (but not specifically by page or line) and in alphabetical order, to make it easier for you to look them up yourself. Following are each chapter's references as well as books, videos, and music I recommend to parents.

Chapter 1: Why Massage Your Baby?
REFERENCES

Adamson, S. "Hands-on therapy." *Health Visitor* 66:2 (February 1993).

———. "Teaching baby massage to new parents." *Complementary Therapies in Nursing and Midwifery* 2:6 (December 1996).

Ainsworth, M. *Infancy in Uganda.* Baltimore: Johns Hopkins University Press, 1967.

Auckett, A. "Baby massage: An alternative to drugs." *Australian Nurses Journal* 9:5 (November 1979).

Barnard, K. E., and Brazelton, T. B., eds. *Touch: The Foundation of Experience.* Madison, WI: International University Press, 1990.

Brown, C., et al., eds. *The Many Facets of Touch.* Johnson & Johnson Pediatric Round Table, no. 10. New York: Elsevier, 1984.

Carpenter, E. *Eskimo Realities.* New York: Holt, Rinehart & Winston, 1973.

Clary, E., et al. "Socialization and situational influences on sustained altruism." *Child Development* 57 (1986).

Crockenberg, S. "Infant irritability, mother responsiveness, and social support influences in the security of infant-mother attachment." *Child Development* 52 (1981).

Curran, F. "Massage: A skill at our fingertips." *Modern Midwife*, July 1996.

Day, L. "Infant massage." *Massage Magazine* 1:5 (1986).

Dellinger-Bavolek, J. "Infant massage: Communicating love through touch." *International Journal of Childbirth Education* 11:4 (December 1996).

Devore, I., et al. *Ethology and Psychiatry*. Toronto: University of Toronto Press, 1974.

Epstein, H. "Phrenoblysis: Special brain and mind growth periods." *Developmental Psychobiology*. New York: Wiley, 1974.

Field, T. "Infant massage." *Zero to Three* 14:2 (1993).

———. "Infant massage." *Journal of Perinatal Education* 3:3 (1994).

———. "Massage therapy for infants and children." *Journal of Developmental and Behavioral Pediatrics* 16:2 (April 1995).

Field, T., Schanberg, S., Scafidi, F., Bauer, C., Vega-Lahr, N., Garcia, R., Nystrom, J., and Kuhn, C. "Tactile/kinesthetic stimulation effects on preterm neonates." *Pediatrics* 77 (May 1986).

Fitzgerald, H., et al. *Child Nurturance: Studies of Development in Non-human Primates*, vol. 3. New York: Putnam, 1982.

Goleman, D. "Patterns of love charted in studies." *New York Times*, September 10, 1985.

Gubernick, D., et al. *Parental Care in Mammals*. New York: Plenum Press, 1981.

Hammett, F. "Studies in the thyroid apparatus: I." *American Journal of Physiology* 56 (1921).

———. "Studies in the thyroid apparatus: V." *Endocrinology* 6 (1921).

Harlow, H. "The nature of love." *American Psychologist* 13 (1958).

———. "Love in infant monkeys." *Scientific American* (June 1959).

Harlow, H., and Harlow, M. "Social deprivation in monkeys." *Scientific American* (November 1962).

Harlow, H., Harlow, M., Dodsworth, R., and Arling, G. "Maternal behavior of rhesus monkeys deprived of mothering and peer association in infancy." *Proceedings of the American Philosophical Society* 110 (1966).

Isherwood, D. "Baby massage groups." *Modern Midwife* 4:2 (February 1994).

Kinzey, W., ed. *The Evolution of Human Behavior: Primate Models*. New York: State University of New York Press, 1987.

Leiderman, L., Tulkin, S., and Rosenfeld, A., eds. *Culture and Infancy: Variations in the Human Experience*. New York: Academic Press, 1977.

McClure (Schneider), V. "Infant massage." *Childbirth Educator* 5:4 (Summer 1986).

Medoff, M. "The gentle benefits of baby massage." *East West Journal* 16:2 (February 1986).

Ottenbacher, K. J., et al. "The effectiveness of tactile stimulation as a form of early intervention: Quantitative evaluation." *Developmental and Behavioral Pediatrics* 8:2 (1987).

Pearce, J. *Magical Child.* New York: Dutton, 1977.

Plotsker-Herman, C. "The gentle art of infant massage." *American Baby Magazine* (March 1986).

Prescott, J. "Pleasure/violence reciprocity theory: The distribution of 49 cultures, relating infant physical affection to adult physical violence." *Futurist*, April 1975.

Queen, S., and Habenstein, R. *The Family in Various Cultures.* New York: Lippincott, 1961.

Reinis, S., and Goldman, J. *The Development of the Brain.* Springfield, IL: Thomas, 1980.

Restak, R. *The Infant Mind.* New York: Doubleday, 1986.

Rheingold, H. *Maternal Behavior in Mammals.* New York: Van Nostrand Reinhold, 1963.

Rice, R. "Neurophysiological development in premature infants following stimulation." *Developmental Psychology* 13 (1977).

Roberts, M. "Baby love." [Effects of infant experience on later adult love life; a study by Shaver and Hazan.] *Psychology Today*, March 1987.

Rorke, L., and Riggs, H. *Myelination of the Brain in the Newborn.* Philadelphia: Lippincott, 1969.

Schneider, E. F. "The power of touch: Massage for infants." *Infants and Young Children* 8:3 (January 1996).

Selye, H. *Stress Without Distress.* New York: New American Library, 1974.

Slater, C. "The effects of tactile stimulation on infants." *Massage Magazine* 28 (1990).

Sullivan, L. E. "The gift of touch." *American Baby Magazine* 57:8 (August 1995).

Trotter, R. "The play's the thing: Baby massage." *Psychology Today*, January 1987.

Whittlestone, W. "The physiology of early attachment in mammals: Implications for human obstetric care." *Medical Journal of Australia* 1 (1978).

Witkin-Lanoil, G. *The Female Stress Syndrome.* New York: Berkley Books, 1984.

Yang, R., et al. "Newborn responses to threshold tactile stimulation." *Child Development* 45:1 (March 1974).

Zborowsky, M., and Herzog, E. *Life Is With People*. New York: International University Press, 1952.

RECOMMENDED BOOKS

Baldwin, R. *Special Delivery*. Berkeley, CA: Celestial Arts, 1979, 1986.

Berends, P. B. *Whole Child, Whole Parent*. New York: Harper, 1975, 1997.

Eisenberg, A., Murkoff, H., and Hathaway, S. *What to Expect the First Year*. New York: Workman Publishing, 1996.

Leach, P. *Babyhood* (revised and expanded). New York: Alfred A. Knopf, 1998.

Leboyer, F. *Loving Hands: The Traditional Art of Baby Massage*. New York: Newmarket, 1976, 1997.

Maiden, A. H., and Farwell, E. *The Tibetan Art of Parenting: From Before Conception Through Early Childhood*. Boston: Wisdom Publications, 1997.

Sears, M., and Sears, W. *25 Things Every New Mother Should Know*. Boston: Harvard Common Press, 1995.

Sears, W., and Sears, M. *The Baby Book: Everything You Need to Know About Your Baby from Birth to Age Two*. New York: Little, Brown, 1993.

Stillerman, E. *Mother Massage: A Handbook for Relieving the Discomforts of Pregnancy*. New York: Dell, 1992.

Chapter 2: Your Baby's Sensory World
REFERENCES

Bernhardt, J. "Sensory capabilities of the fetus." *Maternal Child Nursing* 12 (January–February 1987).

Birnholtz, J. "The development of human fetal eye movement patterns." *Science* 213 (August 7, 1981).

Bower, T. "The visual world of infants." *Scientific American* 215 (December 1966).

Condon, W., and Sander, L. "Neonate movement is synchronized with adult speech: Interactional participation and language acquisition." *Science* 183 (June 1974).

Day, S. "Mother-infant activities as providers of sensory stimulation." *American Journal of Occupational Therapy* 36:9 (December 1982).

DeCasper, A., et al. "Of human bonding: Newborns prefer their mothers' voices." *Science* 208 (June 6, 1980).

Fantz, R. "Maturation of pattern vision in young infants." *Journal of Comparative and Physiological Psychology* 55 (1962).

———. "Pattern vision in newborn infants." *Science* 140 (1963).

Ferreira, A. "Emotional factors in the prenatal environment." *Journal of Nervous and Mental Diseases* 141 (1965).

Figar, W. P., and Moon, C. "Psychobiology of newborn auditory preferences." *Seminars in Perinatology* 13 (1989).

Hooker, D. *The Prenatal Origins of Behavior.* Lawrence, KS: University of Kansas Press, 1952.

Hunziker, U., and Barr, R. "Increased carrying reduces infant crying: A randomized control trial." *Pediatrics* 77 (May 1986).

Kellen, A. "Babies understand 'baby talk,' research suggests." *CNN Interactive*, March 18, 1999.

Klaus, M., and Kennell, J. *Bonding: The Beginning of Parent-Infant Attachment.* New York: New American Library, 1983.

Kuhl, P. 1997, Univ. of Washington: in the article "Goo-goo, Ga-ga Really Helps Baby Learn to Talk," as reported by the Associated Press, CNN Interactive, 7/31/97.

Liley, A. "The fetus as a personality." *Australian and New Zealand Journal of Psychiatry* 6 (1972).

Ludington-Hoe, S., and Golant, S. *How to Have a Smarter Baby.* New York: Rawson Associates, 1985.

McCarthy, P. "Scent: The tie that binds?" *Psychology Today*, July 1986.

Montagu, A. "The skin and human development." *Somatics* 1:3 (Fall 1977).

Pederson, P., et al. "Evidence for olfactory function in utero." *Science* 221 (July 29, 1983).

Porter, R., et al. "The importance of odors in mother-infant interactions." *Maternal Child Nursing* 12 (Fall 1983).

Restak, R. *The Infant Mind.* New York: Doubleday, 1986.

Rowland, R. "Babies learn language lessons before they talk, study shows." *CNN Interactive*, December 31, 1998.

Spence, M., and DeCasper, A. "Prenatal experience with low-frequency maternal voice sounds influences neonatal perception of maternal voice samples." *Infant Behavior and Development* 10 (1987).

Springer, S., and Deutsch, G. *Left Brain, Right Brain.* New York: Freeman, 1985.

Stott. "Children in the womb: Effects of stress." *New Society*, May 19, 1977.

Valman, H., and Pearson, T. "What the fetus feels." *British Medical Journal* 280 (1980).

Verney, T., and Kelly, T. *The Secret Life of the Unborn Child*. New York: Dell, 1981.

Williams, H. Personal interview by author, 1987.

Chapter 3: Bonding, Attachment, and Infant Massage
REFERENCES

Anisfeld, E., Casper, V., Nozyce, M., and Cunningham, N. "Does infant carrying promote attachment? An experimental study of the effects of increased physical contact on the development of attachment." *Child Development* 61 (1990).

Austin, P. "Synchronous movements to human speech." *Perceptual Motor Skills* 79 (1983).

Belsky, J., and Steinberg, L. "The effects of day care: A critical review." *Child Development* 49 (1978).

Bowlby, J. *Attachment and Loss*. New York: Basic Books, 1969, 1996.

Caldwell, B. "The tie that binds: Does daycare weaken the bond with your baby?" *Working Mother*, April 1987.

Capra, F. *The Tao of Physics*. New York: Bantam Books, 1980.

Clary, E., et al. "Socialization and situational influences on sustained altruism." *Child Development* 57 (1986).

Condon, W., and Sander, L. "Neonate movement is synchronized with adult speech: Interactional participation and language acquisition." *Science* 183 (June 1974).

Curry, M. "Maternal attachment behavior and the mother's self-concept: The effect of early skin-to-skin contact." *Nursing Research* 31:2 (March–April 1982).

DeCasper, A., et al. "Of human bonding: Newborns prefer their mothers' voices." *Science* 208 (June 6, 1980).

DeChateau, P., and Wiberg, B. "Long-term effect on mother-infant behavior of extra contact during the first hour postpartum." *Acta Paediatrica* 66 (1977).

Divitto, B., et al. "Talking and sucking: Infant feeding behavior and parent stimulation." *Infant Behavior and Development* 6:2 (April 1983).

D'Spagnat, B. "The quantum theory and reality." *Scientific American*, November 1979.

Edwards, C., et al. "The effects of daycare participation on parent-infant interaction at home." *American Journal of Orthopsychiatry* 57:1 (January 1987).

Fagot, B. I., and Kavanagh, K. "The prediction of antisocial behavior from avoidant attachment classifications." *Child Development* 61 (1990).

Field, T., Guy, L., and Umbel, V. "Infants' responses to mothers' imitative behaviors." *Infant Mental Health Journal* 6:1 (1985).

Grace, M. "Attachment in early childhood." Pact, An Adoption Alliance, 1998. Website: *www.pactadopt.org.*

Harlow, H., and Harlow, M. "Learning to love." *American Scientist* 54 (1959).

————. "Effects of various mother-infant relationships on rhesus monkey behaviors." In *Determinants of Infant Behavior,* edited by B. M. Foss, vol. 4. London: Methuen, 1969.

Hunt, D. *Parents and Children in History.* New York: Basic Books, 1970.

Karen, R. *Becoming Attached: First Relationships and How They Shape Our Capacity to Love.* New York: Oxford University Press, 1998.

Klaus, M., and Kennell, J. *Parent Infant Bonding.* St. Louis: Mosby, 1982.

Lorenz, K. *Evolution and the Modification of Behavior.* Chicago: University of Chicago Press, 1965.

Magid, K., and McKelvey, C. *High Risk: Children Without a Conscience.* New York: Bantam Books, 1987.

McKenna, J. J. *Babies Need Their Mothers Beside Them.* Natural Child Project Society, 1996.

Pearce, J. *Magical Child Matures.* New York: Bantam Books, 1986.

Prescott, J. "Pleasure/violence reciprocity theory: The distribution of 49 cultures, relating infant physical affection to adult physical violence." *Futurist.* (1975, 1985).

Reite, M. "Touch, attachment, and health: Is there a relationship?" In *The Many Facets of Touch,* edited by C. Brown et al., Johnson & Johnson Pediatric Round Table, no. 10. New York: Elsevier, 1984.

Restak, R. *The Infant Mind.* New York: Doubleday, 1986.

Ringler, N., et al. "The effects of extra postpartum contact and maternal speech patterns on children's IQ, speech, and comprehension at five." *Child Development* 49 (1978).

Roberts, M. "Baby love." [Effects of infant experience on later adult love life; study by Shaver and Hazan.] *Psychology Today,* March 1987.

Snow, C. "The development of conversations between mothers and babies." *Journal of Child Language* 4 (1977).

Ziglar, E. "Recommendations of the Yale Bush Center Advisory Committee on Infant Care Leave." *Hearing on parental leave HR 2020 before House Subcommittees on civil service, labor management relations, labor stan-*

dards, and employee benefits (October 17, 1985). Washington, DC: U.S. Government Printing Office, 1985.

RECOMMENDED BOOKS

Brazelton, T. B. *Earliest Relationships: Parents, Infants, and the Drama of Early Attachment.* Reading, MA: Perseus, 1991.

———. *Touchpoints: Your Child's Emotional and Behavioral Development.* Reading, MA: Perseus, 1992.

Briggs, D. C. *Your Child's Self-Esteem.* New York: Doubleday, 1970.

Karen, R. *Becoming Attached: First Relationships and How They Shape Our Capacity to Love.* New York: Oxford University Press, 1998.

Klaus, M., Kennell, J., and Klaus, P. *Bonding: Building the Foundations of Secure Attachment and Independence.* Reading, MA: Perseus, 1996.

Leach, P. *Children First: What Society Must Do—and Is Not Doing—for Children Today.* New York: Random House, 1995.

Liedloff, J. *The Continuum Concept: In Search of Happiness Lost.* Reading, MA: Perseus, 1977, 1998.

Magid, K., and McKelvey, C. *High Risk: Children Without a Conscience.* New York: Bantam Books, 1987.

Pearce, J. *Magical Child.* New York: Dutton, 1977.

———. *Magical Child Matures.* New York: Bantam Books, 1986.

Chapter 4: Especially for Fathers

REFERENCES

Block, J. *Lives Through Time.* Berkeley, CA: Bancroft Books, 1971.

Daly, T. "Men, infant massage, and manhood." *Tender Loving Care.* [Newsletter of the International Association of Infant Massage.] Winter 1987.

DeCasper, A., et al. "Human newborns' perception of male voices: Preference, discrimination, and reinforcing value." *Developmental Psychobiology* 17:5 (September 1984).

Fiefer, M., et al. "A method to help new fathers develop parenting skills." *JOGN Nursing* 10:6 (November–December 1981).

Field, T. "Interaction behaviors of primary versus secondary caretaker fathers." *Developmental Psychology* 14 (1978).

Kennell, J., et al. *Parent Infant Bonding.* St. Louis: Mosby, 1982.

Lamb, M. *The Role of the Father in Child Development.* New York: Wiley, 1981.

Lozoff, M. "Fathers and autonomy in women." In *Women and Success,* edited by R. Kundsin. New York: Morrow, 1974.

Pannabacker, B., et al. "The effect of early extended contact on father-newborn interaction." *Journal of Genetic Psychology* 141 (September 1982).

Parke, R. "Father infant interaction." In *Maternal Attachment and Mothering Disorders*. Johnson & Johnson Pediatric Round Table. New York: Elsevier, 1978.

————. "Father-infant interaction and infant social responsiveness." In *The Handbook of Infant Development*, edited by J. Osofsky. New York: Wiley, 1979.

Taub, D., ed. *Primate Paternalism*. New York: Van Nostrand Reinhold, 1984.

Tuttman. "The father's role in the child's development of the capacity to cope with separation and loss." *Journal of the American Academy of Psychoanalysis*, July 1986.

Zaslow, M., et al. "Depressed mood in fathers: Associations with parent-infant interaction." *Genetic, Social, and General Psychology Monographs* 3:2 (May 1985).

RECOMMENDED BOOKS
Brott, A. *The New Father: A Dad's Guide to the First Year.* New York: Abbeville Press, 1997.

DeMorier, E. *Crib Notes for the First Year of Fatherhood.* Minneapolis: Fairview Press, 1998.

Jamiolkowski, R. *A Baby Doesn't Make the Man: Alternative Sources of Power and Manhood for Young Men.* Teen Pregnancy Prevention Library, 1997.

Karen, R. *Becoming Attached: First Relationships and How They Shape Our Capacity to Love.* New York: Oxford University Press, 1998.

Marzollo, J. *Fathers and Babies: How Babies Grow and What They Need from You, from Birth to Eighteen Months.* New York: HarperCollins, 1993.

Meyer, D., ed. *Uncommon Fathers: Reflections on Raising a Child with a Disability.* Bethesda, MD: Woodbine House, 1995.

Parke, R., Brott, A. *Throwaway Dads: The Myths and Barriers that Keep Men from Being the Fathers They Want to Be.* New York: Houghton Mifflin, 1999.

Chapter 5: Helping Baby (and You) Learn to Relax
REFERENCES
Benson, H., and Proctor, W. *Beyond the Relaxation Response: How to Harness the Healing Power of Your Personal Beliefs.* New York: Berkley, 1994.

Davis, M., et al. *The Relaxation and Stress Reduction Workbook.* New York: New Harbinger, 1998.

Debelle, B. "Relaxation and baby massage." *Australian Nurses Journal* 10:5 (May 1981).

Schaper, K. "Towards a calm baby and relaxed parents." *Family Relations: Journal of Applied Family and Child Studies* 31:3 (July 1982).

Selye, H. *Stress Without Distress.* New York: New American Library, 1974.

RECOMMENDED BOOKS

Benson, H., and Proctor, W. *Beyond the Relaxation Response: How to Harness the Healing Power of Your Personal Beliefs.* New York: Berkley, 1994.

Davis, M., et al. *The Relaxation and Stress Reduction Workbook.* New York: New Harbinger, 1998.

McClure, V. *A Woman's Guide to Tantra Yoga.* Novato, CA: New World Library, 1997.

————. *The Path of Parenting: Twelve Principles to Guide Your Journey.* Novato, CA: New World Library, 1999.

Chapter 6: Music and Massage

REFERENCES

Ayres, B. "Effects of infant carrying practices on rhythm in music." *Ethos* 1:4 (Winter 1973).

Bench, R. "Sound transmission to the human fetus through the maternal abdominal wall." *Journal of Genetic Psychology* 113–14 (1968–69).

Cass-Beggs, B. *Your Baby Needs Music.* New York: St. Martin's Press, 1978.

Daikin, L. *The Lullaby Book.* London: Publications, Ltd., 1959.

Geestesleven, U. *Clump-a-Dump and Snickle-Snack: Pentatonic Songs for Children.* New York: Mercury Press, 1966.

Hill, D., Trehub, S., and Kamenetsky, K. "Mothers' and fathers' songs to infants." *Current Research in Music Cognition,* 1998.

Matterson, E. *This Little Puffin.* London: Penguin Books, 1972.

Opie, I., and Opie, P. *The Oxford Nursery Rhyme Book.* London: Oxford University Press, 1955.

RECOMMENDED BOOKS

Chorao, K. *The Baby's Bedtime Book.* New York: E. P. Dutton, 1984.

Dyer, J. *Animal Crackers: A Delectable Collection of Pictures, Poems, and Lullabies for the Very Young.* New York: Little, Brown, 1996.

Emerson, S., MacLean, C., and MacLean, M. *The Nursery Treasury: A Collection of Baby Games, Rhymes and Lullabies*. New York: Doubleday, 1988.
Kapp, R. *Lullabies: An Illustrated Songbook*. New York: Harcourt Brace, 1997.
McKellar, S. *A Child's Book of Lullabies*. New York: DK Publishing, 1997.

RECOMMENDED MUSIC

Authentic Cajun Lullabies. Mardi Gras CD.
Baby Genius. *Sweet Dream Lullabies*. Imt. Corporation CD.
Beijing Angelic Choir. *Chinese Lullabies*. Wind CD.
Burell, T. *Sweet Baby Lullabies to Soothe Your Newborn*. CD.
Celtic Twilight 3: Lullabies. Hearts of Space CD.
Children's Songs from Around the World, vol. 3: *Lullabies—Asia, Latin America, Africa, Oceania*. Arion CD.
DelRay, M. *Lullabies of Latin America*. WEA/Atlantic/Rhino CD.
Folk Music in Sweden, vol. 6: *Rhymes and Lullabies*. Caprice CD.
Hawaii and Its Lullabies, vol. 20. CD.
Lullabies for Little Angels: Sing Along. Madacy Records CD.
Lullabies: Growing Minds with Music. CD.
N'dege Ocello, M. *Plantation Lullabies*. WEA/Warner Bros. CD.
Palmer, H. *A Child's World of Lullabies*. CD.
Re-Bops, The. *Daddy's Lullabies*. Rebop CD.
Yiddish Lullabies. Israel Music CD.

Chapter 7: Getting Ready

REFERENCES

Daga, et al. "Appropriate technology in keeping babies warm in India." *Annals of Tropical Pediatrics*, March 1986.
Davis, A. *Let's Have Healthy Children*. New York: Harcourt Brace Jovanovich, 1972.
Glas, N. *Conception, Birth, and Early Childhood*. Spring Valley, NY: Anthroposophic Press, 1972.
Johanson, R. B., Spencer, S. A., Rolfe, P., Jones, P., and Massa, D. S. "Effect of post-delivery care on neonatal body temperature." *Acta Paediatrica* 81:11 (November 1992).
Lancet [editorial]. "At what temperature should you keep a baby?" 2:1 (September 12, 1970).
Rutter, N. "Response of term babies to a warm environment." *Archives of the Disabled Child* 53 (March 1979).

Strothers, J., et al. "Thermal balance and sleep state in the newborn infant in a cool environment." *Journal of Physiology* 273 (December 1977).

Wolff, P. "The causes, controls, and organization of behavior in the neonate." *Psychological Issues* [Monograph 17] 5 (1965).

Chapter 8: How to Massage Your Baby
REFERENCES

Berkson, D. *The Foot Book: Healing with the Integrated Treatment of Foot Reflexology.* New York: Funk & Wagnalls, 1977.

Crelin, E. *Functional Anatomy of the Newborn.* New Haven: Yale University Press, 1973.

Chapter 9: Crying, Fussing, and Other Baby Language
REFERENCES

Acredolo, L., and Goodwyn, S. *Baby Signs: How to Talk with Your Baby Before Your Baby Can Talk.* Chicago: Contemporary Books, 1996.

Anisfeld, E., Casper, V., Nozyce, M., and Cunningham, N. "Does infant carrying promote attachment? An experimental study of the effects of increased physical contact on the development of attachment." *Child Development* 61 (1990).

Ainsworth, M., and Bell, S. "Infant crying and maternal responsiveness." *Child Development* 43 (1972).

Chisolm. "Swaddling, cradleboards, and the developing child." *Early Human Development* 2:3 (September 1978).

Crockenberg, S. "Infant irritability, mother responsiveness, and social support influences in the security of infant-mother attachment." *Child Development* 52 (1981).

Cunningham, N., Anisfeld, E., Casper, V., and Nozyce, M. "Infant carrying, breastfeeding, and mother-infant relations: Cache or carry? Experimental evidence for positive effects of early infant carrying." *Lancet* 14 (February 1987).

Gatts, J. D., et al. "Reduced crying and irritability in neonates using a continuously controlled early environment." *Infant Advantage: Clinical Reports*, 1995.

Gray, L., Watt, L., and Blass, E. M. "Skin-to-skin contact is analgesic in healthy newborns." *Pediatrics* 105 #1:e14, January 2000.

Hunziker, U., and Barrm R. "Increased carrying reduces infant crying: A randomized controlled trial." *Pediatrics* 77:5 (May 1986).

Johanson, R. B., Spencer, S. A., Rolfe, P., Jones, P., and Massa, D. S.

"Effect of post-delivery care on neonatal body temperature." *Acta Paediatrica* 81:11 (November 1992).

Kopp, C. "A comparison of stimuli effective in soothing distressed infants." *Dissertation Abstracts* 31:12B (June 1971).

Korner, A., and Thoman, E. "The relative efficacy of contact and vestibular-proprioceptive stimulation on soothing neonates." *Child Development* 43 (1972).

Levy, T. M., and Orlans, M. *Attachment, Trauma, and Healing: Understanding and Treating Attachment Disorder in Children and Families.* Washington, D.C.: CWLA Press, 1998.

Moss, J., et al. "Swaddling, then, there, and now: Historical, anthropological, and current practices." *Maternal Child Nursing* 8:3 (Fall 1979).

Murray, A. "Infant crying as an elicitor of parental behavior." *Psychological Bulletin* 86 (1979).

Roberts, M. "No language but a cry." *Psychology Today*, June 1987.

Sagi, A., and Hoffman, M. "Empathic distress in the newborn." *Developmental Psychology*, 1976.

Sears, W., and Sears, M. *Parenting the Fussy Baby and the High Need Child: Everything You Need to Know from Birth to Age Five.* New York: Little, Brown, 1996.

Shaw, C. "A comparison of the patterns of mother-baby interactions for the group of crying, irritable babies and a group of more amenable babies." *Child Care, Health, and Development* 3 (1977).

Sherman, M. "Differentiation of emotional responses in infants: The ability of observers to judge the emotional characteristics of crying infants." *Journal of Comparative Psychology* 5 (1927).

Simner, M. "Newborn's responses to the cry of another infant." *Developmental Psychology* 5 (1971).

Solter, A. *The Aware Baby: A New Approach to Parenting.* Goleta, CA: Shining Star Press, 1984.

Wipfler, P. *Listening to Children: Crying.* Palo Alto, CA: Parents Leadership Institute, 1990.

RECOMMENDED BOOKS

Jones, S. *Crying Baby, Sleepless Nights.* Boston: Harvard Common Press, 1992.

Sammons, W., and Brazelton, T. B. *The Self-Calmed Baby.* New York: St. Martin's Press, 1991.

Sears, W., and Sears, M. *Parenting the Fussy Baby and the High Need Child: Everything You Need to Know from Birth to Age Five.* New York: Little, Brown, 1996.

Solter, A. *The Aware Baby: A New Approach to Parenting.* Goleta, CA: Shining Star Press, 1984, 1998.

————. *Tears and Tantrums: What to Do When Babies and Children Cry.* Goleta, CA: Shining Star Press, 1998.

Chapter 10: Minor Illness and Colic

REFERENCES

Anderson, G. "Infant colic: A possible solution." *Maternal Child Nursing* 8 (1983).

Barr, R. G., McMullan, S. J., Spiess, H., et al. "Carrying as colic 'therapy': A randomized controlled trial." *Pediatrics* 87 (1991).

Carey, W. "Maternal anxiety and infantile colic: Is there a relationship?" *Clinical Pediatrics* 31 (1968).

Craven, D. "Why colic?" *Medical Journal of Australia* 2 (1979).

Evans, R., et al. "Maternal diet and infantile colic in breastfed infants." *Lancet* 1 (1981).

Hsu, C. Y., et al. "Local massage after vaccination enhances the immunogenicity of diphtheria-tetanus-pertussis vaccine." *Pediatric Infectious Disease Journal* 14:7 (July 1995).

Jakobsson, L., and Lindberg, T. "Cow's milk proteins cause infantile colic in breastfed infants: A double blind study." *Pediatrics* 71 (1983).

Johanson, R. B., Spencer, S. A., Rolfe, P., Jones, P., and Massa, D. S. "Effect of post-delivery care on neonatal body temperature." *Acta Paediatrica* 81:11 (November 1992).

Larsen, J. H. "Infants' colic and belly massage." *Practitioner* 234 (April 1990).

Liebman, W. "Infantile colic: Association with lactose and milk intolerance." *Journal of the American Medical Association* 245 (1981).

Lothe, L., et al. "Cow's milk formula as a cause of infantile colic: A double-blind study." *Pediatrics* 70 (1982).

Paradise, J. "Maternal and other factors in the etiology of infantile colic." *Journal of American Medical Association* 197 (1966).

Said, G., et al. "Clinical trial of the treatment of colic by modification of parent-infant interaction." *Pediatrics* 74 (1984).

Sears, W., and Sears, M. *Parenting the Fussy Baby and the High Need Child: Everything You Need to Know from Birth to Age Five.* New York: Little, Brown, 1996.

Wessel, M., et al. "Paroxysmal fussing in infancy, sometimes called colic." *Pediatrics* 14 (1954).

RECOMMENDED BOOKS

Sears, W., and Sears, M. *Parenting the Fussy Baby and the High Need Child: Everything You Need to Know from Birth to Age Five.* New York: Little, Brown, 1996.

Solter, A. *The Aware Baby: A New Approach to Parenting.* Goleta, CA: Shining Star Press, 1984, 1998.

―――. *Tears and Tantrums: What to Do When Babies and Children Cry.* Goleta, CA: Shining Star Press, 1998.

Chapter 11: Your Premature Baby

REFERENCES

Affleck, G., Tennen, J. H., and Rowe, J. "Mothers, fathers, and the crisis of newborn intensive care." *Infant Mental Health Journal* 11:1 (1990).

Anisfeld, E., Casper, V., Nozyce, M., and Cunningham, N. "Does infant carrying promote attachment? An experimental study of the effects of increased physical contact on the development of attachment." *Child Development* 61 (1990).

Dunn, C., Sleep, J., and Collett, D. "Sensing an improvement: An experimental study to evaluate the use of aromatherapy, massage and periods of rest in an intensive care unit." *Journal of Advanced Nursing* 21:1 (January 1995).

Field, T. "Interventions for premature infants." *Journal of Pediatrics* 109 (1986).

Field, T., Schanberg, S., Gunzenhauser, N., and Brazelton, T. "Massage stimulates growth in preterm infants: A replication." *Infant Behavior and Development* 13 (1990).

Field, T., Schanberg, S., Scafidi, F., Bauer, C., Vega-Lahr, N., Garcia, R., Nystrom, J., and Kuhn, C. "Cardiac and behavioral responses to repeated tactile and auditory stimulation of preterm and term neonates." *Developmental Psychology* 15 (July 1979).

―――. "Tactile/kinesthetic stimulation effects on preterm neonates." *Pediatrics* 77 (May 1986).

Gottfried, A., et al. "Touch as an organizer for learning and development." In *The Many Facets of Touch*, edited by C. Brown et al. Johnson & Johnson Pediatric Round Table, no. 10. New York: Elsevier, 1980.

Grossman, K., et al. "Maternal tactual contact of the newborn after various postpartum conditions of mother-infant contact." *Developmental Psychology* 17 (March 1981).

Harrison, L. L., Leeper, J., and Yoon, M. "Effects of gentle human touch on preterm infants: Results from a pilot study." *Infant Behavior and Development* 15 (1990).

———. "Early parental touch and preterm infants." *JOGN Nursing* 20:4 (1991).

———. "Effects of hospital-based instruction on interactions between parents and preterm infants." *Neonatal Network* 9:7 (1991).

———. "Preterm infants' physiologic responses to early parent touch." *Western Journal of Nursing Research* 13:6 (1991).

Harrison, L. L., et al. "Effects of gentle human touch on preterm infants: Results from a pilot study." *Infant Behavior and Development* 15 (1992).

Heffernan, A., et al. "Baby massage—a teaching model." *Australian Nurses Journal* 13:6 (December–January 1984).

Heller, S. A. "A comparison of the effects of containment and stroking of preterm infants at varying levels of maturity." Ph.D. diss. Chicago: Loyola University of Chicago, 1991.

Johanson, R. B., Spencer, S. A., Rolfe, P., Jones, P., and Massa, D. S. "Effect of post-delivery care on neonatal body temperature." *Acta Paediatrica* 81:11 (November 1992).

Klaus, M., and Fanaroff, A. *Care of the High-risk Neonate.* Philadelphia: Saunders, 1986.

Kramer, M., et al. "Extra tactile stimulation of the premature infant." *Nursing Research* 24 (September–October 1975).

Kuhn, C. M., et al. "Tactile-kinesthetic stimulation effects on sympathetic and adrenocortical function in preterm infants." *Journal of Pediatrics* 119:3 (1991).

McGrade, B. J., Affleck, G., Alen, D., and McQueeney, M. "Mothers of high-risk infants: Is their initial use of early intervention a predictor of later coping?" *Infant Mental Health Journal* 6:1 (1985).

McIntosh, N. "Massage in preterm infants." *Archives of Disease in Childhood Fetal and Neonatal Education* 70:1 (January 1994).

Moses, H., and Phillips, R. "Skin hunger effects on preterm neonates." *Infant-Toddler Intervention* 6:1 (1996).

Oehler, J. "The development of the preterm infant's responsiveness to auditory and tactile social stimuli." *Dissertation Abstracts* 45:8B (February 1985).

Paterson, L. "Baby massage in the neonatal unit." *Nursing: Journal of Clinical Practice, Education and Management* [London] 4:23 (November–December 1990).

Powell, L. "The effect of extra stimulation and maternal involvement on the development of low birthweight infants and on maternal behavior." *Child Development* 45 (March 1974).

Rausch, P. "Effects of tactile and kinesthetic stimulation on premature infants." *JOGN Nursing* 10:1 (1981).

―――. "A tactile and kinesthetic stimulation program for premature infants." In *The Many Facets of Touch*, edited by C. Brown et al. Johnson & Johnson Pediatric Round Table, no. 10. New York: Elsevier, 1984.

Rice, R. "Premature infants respond to sensory stimulation." *APA Monitor*, November 1975.

―――. "Cardiac and behavioral responsivity to tactile stimulation in premature and full term infants." *Developmental Psychology* 12:4 (July 1976).

―――. "Neurophysiological development in premature infants following stimulation." *Developmental Psychology* 13 (1977).

Rose, S. "Effects of prematurity and early intervention on responsivity to tactual stimuli: A comparison of term and preterm infants." *Child Development* 51:2 (June 1980).

―――. "Preterm responses to passive, active, and social touch." In *The Many Facets of Touch*, edited by C. Brown et al. Johnson & Johnson Pediatric Round Table, no. 10. New York: Elsevier, 1984.

Scafidi, F., et al. "Effects of tactile/kinesthetic stimulation on the clinical course and sleep/wake behavior of preterm neonates." *Infant Behavior and Development* 9:1 (January 1986).

―――. "Massage stimulates growth in preterm infants: A replication." *Infant Behavior and Development* 13 (1990).

Schaeffer, J. "The effects of gentle human touch on mechanically ventilated very short gestation infants." *Maternal Child Nursing* [Monograph 12], vol. 11 (1982).

Stern, M., et al. "Prematurity stereotyping: Effects on mother-infant interaction." *Child Development* 57:2 (April 1986).

Walt, J., et al. "Mother-infant interactions at two and three months in preterm, SGA, and full term infants." *Early Human Development*, September 1985.

White, J., et al. "The effects of tactile and kinesthetic stimulation on neonatal development in the premature infant." *Developmental Psychobiology* 9 (November 1976).

White-Traut, R. C., and Goldman, M. N. "Maternally administered tactile, auditory, visual and vestibular stimulation: Relationship to later interactions between mothers and premature infants." *Research in Nursing and Health* 11 (1988).

RECOMMENDED BOOKS
Harrison, H. *The Premature Baby Book.* New York: St. Martin's Press, 1978, 1983.

Klein, A. H., and Ganon, J. A. *Caring for Your Premature Baby.* New York: HarperCollins, 1998.

Ludington-Hoe, S., and Golant, S. *Kangaroo Care: The Best You Can Do for Your Preterm Infant.* New York: Bantam Books, 1996.

Manginello, F. P., Foy, T., and DiGeroniomo, M., eds. *Your Premature Baby.* New York: John Wiley & Sons, 1998.

Chapter 12: Your Baby with Special Needs
REFERENCES
Als, H., et al. "Stages of early behavioral organization: The study of a sighted infant and a blind infant in interaction with their mothers." In *High Risk Infants and Children, Adult and Peer Interactions.* New York: Academic Press, 1980.

Ayres, J. *Sensory Integration and the Child.* Los Angeles: Western Psychological Services, 1979.

Bigelow, A. "The development of reaching in blind infants." *British Journal of Developmental Psychology* 4 (November 1988).

Bushnell, E. "Relationship between visual and tactual exploration by six-month-olds." *Developmental Psychology* 21:4 (July 1985).

Clark, L. "The importance of touch with an anencephalic baby." *Maternal Child Nursing* 7:5 (September–October 1982).

Cratty, B., and Sams, T. *The Body Image of Blind Children.* New York: American Foundation for the Blind, 1968.

Drehobl, K., and Fuhr, M., *Pediatric Massage for the Child with Special Needs.* Tucson: Therapy Skill Builders, 1991.

Fraser, B. "Child Impairment and Parent-Infant Communication." *Child Care, Health, and Development* 12 (1986).

Gregory, S. "Mother speech to young hearing impaired children." *Journal of the British Association of Teachers of the Deaf* 3 (1979).

Hansen, R. "Motorically impaired infants: Impact of a massage procedure on caregiver-infant interactions." *Journal of the Multi-Handicapped Person* 1:1 (1988).

Harrison, H. *The Premature Baby Book.* New York: St. Martin's Press, 1983.

Hart, V. "Characteristics of young blind children." Paper presented at the Second International Symposium on Visually Handicapped Infants and Young Children: Birth to Seven. Aruba, 1983.

Infant Hearing Resource. *Parent-Infant Communication: A Program of Clinical and Home Training for Parents and Hearing Impaired Infants.* Portland, OR: Infant Hearing Resource, 1985.

Korner, A., et al. "Visual alertness in neonates as evoked by maternal care." *Journal of Experimental Child Psychology* 10 (1970).

Linkous, L. W. "Passive tactile stimulation effects on the muscle tone of hypotonic, developmentally delayed young children." *University of Alabama* (1990).

Porter, S. J. "The use of massage for neonates requiring special care." *Complementary Therapies in Nursing and Midwifery,* August 1996.

Riesen, A. "Sensory Deprivation." In *Progress in Physiological Psychology,* edited by E. Stellar and J. Sprague. New York: Academic Press, 1966.

Scafidi, F., and Field, T. "Massage therapy improves behavior in neonates born to HIV-positive mothers." *Journal of Pediatric Psychology* 21:6 (December 1996).

Simons, R. *After the Tears: Parents Talk About Raising a Child with a Disability.* Denver, CO: Children's Museum of Denver, 1985.

Slater, C. "Massaging crack babies." *Massage Magazine* 28 (1990).

Speirer, J. *Infant Massage for Developmentally Delayed Babies.* Denver, CO: United Cerebral Palsy Center, 1982.

———. *Therapeutic Infant Massage as an Intervention for Parent and Child Attachment.* Denver, CO: United Cerebral Palsy Center, 1982.

Strauss, L. "The effects of tactile stimulation on the communicative, social-emotional, and motor behaviors of deaf-blind-multi-handicapped infants." *Dissertation Abstracts* 42:10A (April 1982).

Warren, D. *Blindness and Early Childhood Development.* New York: American Foundation for the Blind, 1984.

Weber, K. "Massage for drug exposed infants." *Massage Therapy Journal,* 1991.

Wheeden, A., Scafidi, F. A., Field, T., Ironson, G., Valdeon, C., and Band-stra, E, "Massage effects on cocaine-exposed preterm neonates." *Journal of Developmental and Behavioral Pediatrics* 14:5 (1993).

White, B., and Held, R. "Plasticity of sensorimotor development in the human infant." In *Causes of Behavior: Readings in Child Development and Educational Psychology*, 2d ed., edited by J. Rosenblith, and W. Allinsmith. Boston: Allyn & Bacon, 1966.

Wills, D. "The ordinary devoted mother and her blind baby." *Psychoanalytic Study of the Child* 34 (1979).

Zimmerman, J. "Social interaction patterns between blind and multi-impaired infants and their mothers: An analysis." *Dissertation Abstracts* 42:7A (1982).

RECOMMENDED BOOKS

Behrman, R. E. *The Future of Children: Drug Exposed Infants.* New York: Center for the Future of Children, 1991.

Bull, M. T. *Keys to Parenting a Child with Down Syndrome.* New York: Barrons, 1993.

Geralis, E., ed. *Children with Cerebral Palsy: A Parent's Guide.* Bethesda, MD: Woodbine House, 1998.

Holbrook, M., ed. *Children with Visual Impairments: A Parent's Guide.* Bethesda, MD: Woodbine House, 1996.

Hughes, S. *What Makes Ryan Tick: A Family's Triumph over Tourette Syndrome and Attention Deficiency Hyperactivity Disorder.* Carol Stream, IL: Hope Press, 1996.

Kephart, B. *A Slant of Sun: One Child's Courage.* New York: W.W. Norton, 1998.

Kranowitz, C., and Silver, L. *The Out-of-Sync Child: Recognizing and Coping with Sensory Integration Dysfunction.* New York: Perigee, 1998.

Meyer, D. J., ed. *Uncommon Fathers: Reflections on Raising a Child with a Disability.* Bethesda, MD: Woodbine House, 1995.

Miller, F., and Bachrach, S. J. *Cerebral Palsy: A Complete Guide for Caregiving.* Baltimore: Johns Hopkins University Press, 1995.

Ogden, P. W. *The Silent Garden: Raising Your Deaf Child.* Washington, D.C.: Gallaudet University Press, 1982.

Sacks, O. *Seeing Voices: A Journey into the World of the Deaf.* New York: Harper, 1990.

Shapiro, L. *Uncommon Voyage: Parenting a Special Needs Child in the World of Alternative Medicine.* London: Faber and Faber, 1997.

Simons, R. *After the Tears: Parents Talk about Raising a Child with a Disability.* New York: Harcourt Brace, 1991.

Stray-Gundersen, K. *Babies with Down Syndrome: A New Parent's Guide.* Bethesda, MD: Woodbine House, 1995.

Sumar, S. *Yoga for the Special Child: A Therapeutic Approach for Infants and Children with Down Syndrome, Cerebral Palsy, and Learning Disabilities.* Buckingham, NY: Special Yoga Publications, 1998. Website: *http://www.specialyoga.com.* E-mail: *Info@specialyoga.com.*

Chapter 13: Your Growing Child

REFERENCES

Karen, R. *Becoming Attached: First Relationships and How They Shape Our Capacity to Love.* New York: Oxford University Press, 1998.

Montague, A. *Touching.* New York: Harper and Row, 1978.

Zacher-Laves, C. U. "Suggestions for adaptations of the massage with the growing child." Private communication to author, 1999.

RECOMMENDED BOOKS

Cole, J., Calmenson, S., and Tiegreen, A. *Pat-a-Cake and Other Play Rhymes.* New York: Morrow, 1992.

Cole, J., Tiegreen, A., and Calmenson, S. *The Eentsy, Weentsy Spider: Finger-plays and Action Rhymes.* New York: Morrow, 1991.

Staff, T., and Mohrmann, G. *1001 Rhymes and Fingerplays.* Boston: Watten Publishing House, 1994.

Chapter 14: Your Adopted or Foster Children

REFERENCES

Acredolo, L., and Goodwyn, S. *Baby Signs: How to Talk to Your Baby Before Your Baby Can Talk.* Chicago: Contemporary Books, 1996.

Bond, J. "Post adoption depression syndrome." *Roots and Wings.* ADOPT: Assistance Information Support (Spring 1995). Website: *www.adopting.org/pads.html.*

Clark, S. "Prenatal trauma and the adoptee experience." San Francisco: Pact, An Adoption Alliance, 1998. Website: *www.pactadopt.org.*

Dubucs, R. "Touching and the adopted child." *International Concerns for Children* (1998).

Grace, M. "Attachment in early childhood." San Francisco: Pact, An Adoption Alliance, 1998. Web site: *www.pactadopt.org.*

Hage, D. "Foundations of attachment." *International Concerns for Children* (1999).

Henning, R. S. Personal letter to author, 1999.

Ingram, J. "Russian foster families face huge task." *Philadelphia Inquirer,* December 18, 1998.

Karen, R. *Becoming Attached: First Relationships and How They Shape Our Capacity to Love.* New York: Oxford University Press, 1998.

Kurson, B. "Foster parents face a life of tough breaks." *Chicago Sun Times,* March 14, 1999.

Melina, L. "Attachment to older child has some twists." *Adopted Child,* January 1985.

———. "Unattached child: Going through life not caring." *Adopted Child* (February 1985).

———. "Attachment theorists believe parent-infant experiences determine later behavior." *Adopted Child,* May 1997.

Russell, M. "The lifelong impact of adoption." San Francisco: Pact, An Adoption Alliance, 1998. Website: *www.pactadopt.org.*

Singer, L., et al. "Mother-infant attachment in adoptive families." *Child Development* 56 (December 1985).

Steinberg, G. "Bonding and attachment: How does adoption affect a newborn?" San Francisco: Pact, An Adoption Alliance, 1998. Website: *www.pactadopt.org.*

"The Special Love of Foster Parents." *Record Online* (December 6, 1998).

Verrier, N. "Healing the primal wound." San Francisco: PACT, An Adoption Alliance, 1998. Website: *www.pactadopt.org.*

RECOMMENDED BOOKS

Babb, L., Laws, R., and DeBolt, R. *Adopting and Advocating for the Special Needs Child.* Bergin & Garvey, 1997.

Davis, S. *Do You Want to Be a Foster Parent?* Lucid Press, 1998.

Karen, R. *Becoming Attached: First Relationships and How They Shape Our Capacity to Love.* New York: Oxford University Press, 1998.

Melina, L. *Raising Adopted Children.* New York: HarperPerennial, 1998.

Russell, M. *Adoption Wisdom: A Guide to the Issues and Feelings of Adoption.* Boston: Broken Branch Productions, 1996.

Verrier, N. *The Primal Wound: Understanding the Adopted Child.* 1993.

Chapter 15: A Note to Teen Parents
REFERENCES

Crockenberg, S. B. "Professional support for adolescent mothers: Who gives it, how adolescent mothers evaluate it, what they would prefer." *Infant Mental Health Journal* 4:1 (1986).

Field, T., Widmayer, S., Adler, S., and de Cubas, M. *Teenage Parenting in Different Cultures, Family Constellations, and Caregiving Environments: Effects on Infant Development.* Miami: University of Miami Medical School, 1986.

Herzog, E. P., Cherniss, D. S., and Menzel, B. J. "Issues in engaging high-risk adolescent mothers in supportive work." *Infant Mental Health Journal* 7:1 (1986).

Karen, R. *Becoming Attached: First Relationships and How They Shape Our Capacity to Love.* New York: Oxford University Press, 1998.

RECOMMENDED BOOKS

Gore, A. *The Hip Mama Survival Guide.* New York: Hyperion, 1998.

Jamiolkowski, R. *A Baby Doesn't Make the Man: Alternative Sources of Power and Manhood for Young Men.* Teen Pregnancy Prevention Library, 1997.

Lerman, E., and Moffett, J. *Teen Moms: The Pain and the Promise.* Buena Park, CA: Morning Glory Press, 1997.

Simpson, C. *Coping with Teenage Motherhood.* NY: Rosen Publishing Group, 1997.

Trapani, M. *Listen Up: Teenage Mothers Speak Out.* NY: Rosen Publishing Group, 1997.

RESOURCES

I appreciate comments and questions from my readers. I can also be reached through my publisher.

International Association of Infant Massage
Founder: Vimala McClure
E-mail: vimalaji@comcast.net
Blogs: http://spiritual-parents.blogspot.com
http://intuitive-parents.blogspot.com

International Association of Infant Massage
E-mail: iaiminfo@gmail.com

United States Association
Website: www.infantmassageusa.org

For chapters of IAIM outside the United States, please contact the international office. We are growing quickly all over the world, and there will be many more instructors, trainers, and websites as the years pass. Most chapters and instructor trainers have e-mail addresses or fax numbers, and the international office should be able to give them to you. If not, contact the U.S. chapter office or me.

Many of the CIMIs (certified infant massage instructors) in the IAIM have developed specialized programs, videos, and Websites, offering a wide range of help in this area.

A word of caution: Just because someone is a massage therapist does not mean they know how to teach infant massage. Be cautious about programs offered on-line. Some massage therapists think they can make up a series of strokes and then teach them as infant massage. But the ancient art of infant massage is not at all like adult massage, and it is not another "playtime" exercise. You must know not only how a baby's body works but the significance of the relationship between the caregiver and the baby, the way the baby's responses change as he or she grows, what a baby's cues mean, and many other subtle aspects of parent-infant communication, to properly teach infant massage. Babies do not respond well to poking, tickling, or deep tissue work, or to massage that is too tentative and light.

Special babies with special needs also need a special way of being massaged. All babies must be followed in their growth periods and responded to with respect, genuineness, and above all love. The infant massage we teach is based on the idea that massage is one of the best tools we have to continue the attachment process, and so how we massage the baby, and how we respond to the baby's communication, is very important.

The massage we teach is thousands of years old, proven in the laboratory of human experience. The routine I developed is based on age-old practices, put together in a way that works. I named and organized most of the strokes to be of best benefit to most babies and I created the Colic Relief Routine, Touch Relaxation, and many other aspects of what is in this book, so it is easy for me to see whether someone has been trained in our program or made up their own. Of course, as you get to know your baby and learn the program, you will find your own ways of massaging your baby that are just right for you. But I believe it is important before improvising to first get the instruction properly from an IAIM certified instructor. In this way, your improvisations will benefit and not possibly harm your little one.

The thousands of parents who have received our instruction since 1976 would echo these cautions. Most say they never realized how deep and profound the experience was until they had finished a class series. Where your baby is concerned, nothing but the best should be your guide.

United States Websites and Programs by Certified Infant Massage Instructor Trainers:

Maria Mathias Infant Massage Programs
(Maria Mathias, CIMI and instructor trainer, New Mexico)
Maria also has special continuing education programs for medically
    fragile infants.
E-mail: waynem1@flash.net
Website: http://www.infantmassageinstitute.com

Bonding and Relaxation Techniques (BART)
(Evelyn Guyer, CIMI and instructor trainer, New York)
Evelyn also specializes in special needs populations.
E-mail: EGUYER@aol.com

DeAnna Wamsley Elliott
(CIMI and instructor trainer, Colorado)
DeAnna also specializes in prenatal and early birth imprinting.
E-mail: elliott@amigo.net

Helena Moses
(CIMI and instructor trainer, Florida)
Helena also specializes in premature and at-risk babies.
E-mail: helena m@juno.com

Juliana Bavolek
(CIMI and instructor trainer, North Carolina)
Juliana also specializes in at-risk families and teen parents.
E-mail: JulianaDB@aol.com

Audrey Downes
(CIMI and instructor trainer, California)
Audrey also helped found the IAIM and is active in its management.
E-mail: ddownes@ecst.csuchico.edu

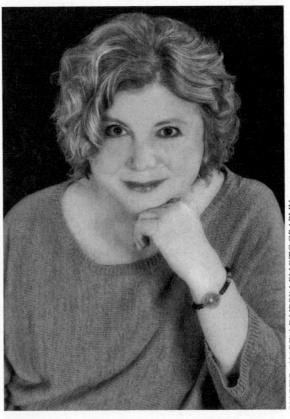

ABOUT THE AUTHOR

VIMALA MCCLURE lives in Boulder, Colorado, her "ancestral home." She has been practicing yoga and meditation since 1970 and taught yoga for several years before giving birth to her two children, now adults. Vimala then turned her attention to the world of parenting, and after spending time serving in an orphanage in northern India, Vimala brought the age-old practice of infant massage to the West in her groundbreaking first book, *Infant Massage: A Handbook for Loving Parents*. For several years, she taught parents the art of infant massage out of her home. In 1978, at the request of childbirth educators, she developed a training program and began to train instructors to teach the program she had developed in India, incorporating Swedish and reflexology methods and yoga postures and poses adapted for babies. She named the strokes, designed a special routine for colicky babies, and developed a course for parents that became the core curriculum for her upcoming organization. After several years, she trained a group of instructors to train other instructors, and the International Association of Infant Massage was born, incorporated as a nonprofit organization in 1986. The IAIM now has more than twenty-seven chapters worldwide, and her book has been translated into many languages. Vimala was able to travel to India many times during these years, and she had the great fortune of working in Mother Teresa's Shishu Bhavan (baby hospital) in Calcutta. Since then, Vimala has continued to write for many magazines and has authored several more books. Now that her children are grown, she also has time to pursue fiber arts and has become an award-winning quilt artist. Vimala continues to write about parenting and quiltmaking and to produce her works of fiber art.